UNCONVENTIONAL MEDICINE

UNCONVENTIONAL MEDICINE

JOIN THE REVOLUTION TO REINVENT HEALTHCARE, REVERSE CHRONIC DISEASE, AND CREATE A PRACTICE YOU LOVE

CHRIS KRESSER

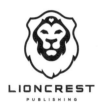

LIONCREST
PUBLISHING

UNCONVENTIONAL MEDICINE
Join the Revolution to Reinvent Healthcare, Reverse
Chronic Disease, and Create a Practice You Love

ISBN   978-1-61961-747-6 *Paperback*
         978-1-61961-748-3 *Ebook*

CONTENTS

FOREWORD

BY MARK HYMAN, MD

"So, what is disease? In old times people used to think that a disease was some actual entity or thing which had got into the body in some way, and was there lying hidden and secreted, and was to be cast out. This idea, which we now know to be true only in a few specific instances, was at one time general. ... The conclusion is that all disease is disordered function. Here, then, I say, is the highest justification for all treatment being based upon the principle of restoring disordered functions to order, and this is what I have ventured to term Functional Medicine."

WILLOUGHBY F. WADE, BA, MB,

PHYSICIAN TO THE GENERAL HOSPITAL,

BIRMINGHAM, ENGLAND

DELIVERED AS A CLINICAL LECTURE ON

FUNCTIONAL MEDICINE, MARCH 5, 1870

PUBLISHED IN THE JULY 1, 1871 ISSUE OF *THE LANCET*

When I graduated from medical school I believed I had the keys to the kingdom, that I knew everything there was to know about medicine and healing. If I didn't learn it in medical school, it was either not scientific or worse, harmful. I believed I could help all my patients by applying what I learned. And yes, I could help people with acute illness, but the bulk of my country family practice patients had chronic illnesses that were mostly preventable and reversible. I felt like I was working for Pharma.

Then I became ill with chronic fatigue syndrome, and medicine provided no answers. It was only when I listened to Dr. Jeffrey Bland that I realized there was a different way of thinking about disease, a different paradigm based on understanding the body as an integrated system, a model based on analysis of root causes of disease. I said to myself, "Either this man is crazy, or what he is saying is true." And if it is true, then I owe it to myself and my patients to explore the model. I did and cured myself of mercury toxicity that resulted from living in China.

I began using the model on my patients, with often extraordinary results. Twenty years later and tens of thousands of patients later, I know this is the future of medicine—both from a scientific perspective and to help physicians become re-enchanted with medicine. Now, I run Cleveland Clinic Center for Functional Medicine with over fifty employees in a 17,000-square-foot space in the epicenter of Cleveland Clinic. We are doing research and education, as well as community- and group-based programs.

Many of you may be disillusioned with traditional medical practice and may be curious about Functional Medicine— one of the approaches that Chris will be discussing at length in this book.

Functional Medicine is a comprehensive theoretical framework for medicine that incorporates a modern understanding of the body as a complex adaptive system, an integrated biological ecosystem, an interdependent, web-like network of biological functions. It provides a new set of lenses through which to interpret and organize complex biological and social information so that we understand much better why we get sick and how we heal. Functional Medicine guides the clinician to a more comprehensive view of the whole organism, not just organs—the whole system, not just the symptoms.

Functional Medicine also provides a practical clinical framework for how the body's physiologic systems are linked together and how their functions are influenced by both environment (diet, lifestyle, microbes, allergens, environmental toxins, and stresses) and genetics (Loscalzo et al. 2007). Applied in practice, it can more effectively prevent, treat, and often cure chronic conditions, at lower cost, through a new way of seeing disease based on underlying causes, and by developing treatment models that can restore balance within dysfunctional biological systems and networks.

A classic patient story highlights the failure of our current model and the power of Functional Medicine to solve complex chronic illness. At fifty-seven, the patient described himself as in general good health and was eager to climb Kilimanjaro. He took fifteen different medications for his colitis, asthma, alopecia areata (total hair loss), and hypertension. He was well treated by an internist, gastroenterologist, pulmonologist, and dermatologist, all of whom made the correct "diagnosis" for each discrete disease based on symptoms (not causes) and provided the appropriate medications for the symptoms or diagnosis. All of his "diseases" were inflammatory in nature, but no physician had investigated the underlying cause of the systemic inflammation that was manifesting in so many ways. Clearly, knowing the names for all his diseases did not help him get better or provide a path to understanding the root causes.

A Functional Medicine work-up that looked at common underlying pathways of disease and dysfunction revealed that each of this patient's diagnoses could be explained by the inflammation caused by something he was eating—gluten. Tests confirmed the diagnosis of celiac disease, which had been missed for more than forty years. Within six months, he was off most of his medications, had lost twenty-five pounds, his blood pressure had improved, he had no more asthma symptoms, he had normal bowel movements, and his hair was growing back. A review in the *New England Journal of Medicine* (Farrell 2002) cataloged the myriad diseases that can be caused by celiac disease, from anemia to osteoporosis, from autoimmune diseases to thyroid dysfunction, from schizophrenia to psoriasis. Because each of these conditions may be triggered by multiple factors, not just eating gluten, consideration of him as a unique individual was critical. His genetics required that he not eat a specific food protein to maintain health, while another patient with the same "disease" might need an entirely different treatment.

Clinical medicine can shift to applied systems medicine—personalized, predictive, preventative, and participatory (Snyderman and Langheier 2006). Most chronic disease is preventable, and much of it is reversible, if a comprehensive, individualized approach addressing genetics, diet, nutrition, environmental exposures, stress, exercise, and psycho-spiritual needs is implemented through integrated clinical teams based on emerging research (ACPM 2009).

I know that you are likely at a crossroads, and are considering or have started shifting your practice and career. I can only say that Chris Kresser's approach in *Unconventional Medicine* is your roadmap to a new and reinvigorated love for medicine.

MARCH 17, 2017

MARK HYMAN, MD

CHAIRMAN, INSTITUTE FOR FUNCTIONAL MEDICINE

DIRECTOR, CLEVELAND CLINIC CENTER
FOR FUNCTIONAL MEDICINE

PART ONE

THE PROMISE

CHAPTER ONE

LEO'S STORY: A CALL TO ACTION

About two years ago, I spoke with the mother of an eight-year-old boy I've been treating—we'll call him Leo. When they first came to me, both of Leo's parents were nearly in tears. They were at their wits' end. Several times a day, Leo would throw epic tantrums for the slightest of reasons. He would end up writhing on the floor, screaming and crying inconsolably. This would happen with something as simple as trying to put shoes on as they were leaving the house, or not cutting the crusts off the bread for his sandwich in just the right way, or getting a stain on one of his favorite t-shirts.

He ate only a handful of foods, nearly all of them processed and refined, like crackers, waffles, and bread. His parents were concerned about nutrient deficiency and the effects of such a limited diet, but each time they tried to introduce new foods, he went crazy. They were completely worn down and didn't have the internal resources to battle him at every meal.

Leo was also extremely rigid about certain self-imposed rules and behavior and his environment. Everything had to be just right. If something in his room was out of place, his toys weren't arranged in just the right order, or the desks in his classroom were not arranged in perfect lines, he'd fly off the handle (his mom often had to come pick him up from school early as a result). This was also true in unfamiliar environments, which made it difficult for them to be away from home for more than a few hours, much less travel or take vacations.

They took Leo to see several doctors locally. He was initially diagnosed on the autism spectrum, but eventually the specialists decided that he more likely had sensory processing disorder and obsessive compulsive disorder.

At first his parents were somewhat relieved to have a diagnosis for Leo. They soon realized, however, that these diagnoses weren't much more than labels for the symptoms Leo experienced. And when they asked the doctors what the treatment was, you can guess the answer: medication.

Leo's parents weren't happy about the idea of medicating their son, but they also saw how much he was suffering and hoped that the drugs would give him some relief. So, they initially tried Adderall, as the doctor suggested. Although Leo did improve slightly in some ways, he developed intractable constipation, sleep problems, headache, and stomach pain. The doctor switched him to Ritalin, but the results were largely the same.

From here, the specialist suggested a selective serotonin reuptake inhibitor (SSRI), which is sometimes used to treat sensory processing disorder. Again, it did help, to some extent, and Leo tolerated it better than Ritalin and Adderall. But as Leo's mother read more online about the potential risks of SSRIs in children and adolescents, she became increasingly uncomfortable about him taking one.

Throughout this entire time, not one of the specialists they consulted even *hinted* that there might be an underlying cause that was contributing to Leo's problems, or suggested anything other than a lifetime of stimulant or antidepressant drugs for treatment. This isn't an exception—it is the norm. Most doctors, and by extension patients and the public, have no idea that mental and behavioral disorders can have physiological causes.

From Old Paradigm to New

Fortunately, one of Leo's mother's friends had read several articles on my blog about the "gut-brain axis" and the connection between inflammation and mental health disorders. She forwarded them to Leo's mom, who then made an appointment with me.

I could tell Leo's parents were a little skeptical when we first met, but after I explained the science behind these links, and shared some stories of other similar patients I'd treated and the results we'd had, they were excited to move forward. So, I ran a complete panel of tests to screen for nutrient deficiency, GI pathologies, blood sugar imbalance, heavy metal toxicity, and food intolerances.

Not surprisingly, I found several issues. Leo had a disrupted gut microbiome, with low levels of beneficial bacteria and high levels of pathogenic microbes. He had gluten intolerance, with possible celiac disease, and he was also intolerant of rice, buckwheat, and corn—which were the major ingredients in the toaster waffles that he ate for dinner daily. He had deficiencies of several nutrients, including B12, folate, iron, and vitamin D. And he showed high levels of arsenic, a heavy metal with toxic effects. Rice milk was the only beverage he would drink aside from water, and it has been shown to be one of the highest dietary sources of arsenic.

We immediately began addressing these issues. Within two weeks, Leo's parents noticed a significant difference in his behavior. He was having fewer tantrums and didn't seem bothered by some of the things that would typically send him into a tailspin.

About six weeks into the treatment, Leo's mom received a call from school. His teacher said, "Who is this kid you're sending to school in place of Leo? I don't even recognize him." Leo's teacher had really struggled with his behavior, just as his parents had, and she was amazed at the difference. He was much more relaxed in the classroom, which was a life-altering change for everyone involved.

When I next talked to Leo's mom, it was about three months into the treatment. We had the follow-up test results back, and many of the initial issues we set out to address—like the disrupted gut microbiome and nutrient deficiencies—were resolved. And according to Leo's mom, Leo was literally a different person. They could hardly believe the changes that they'd observed in the last three months.

His diet had expanded significantly. He was eating things he would have thrown against the wall just a few months before; he was more tolerant of disorder; he was more affectionate and less argumentative, and he was far less bothered by the things that used to trigger inconsolable tantrums that would last for hours.

At the end of our call, his mom said something that really struck me. She asked, "Why don't more doctors know about this approach? There are so many other kids out there like Leo, and their parents and doctors aren't even thinking about the stuff we've worked on here."

Her question is exactly what inspired me to write this book, and to devote my life to training practitioners in the approach we'll be discussing in the following chapters.

My Question for You—and an Opportunity

Her question also represents an opportunity for you: to help the millions of people who, like Leo, are suffering tremendously, but not finding answers in the conventional medical system; an opportunity to break through the old paradigm of disease management and symptom suppression with drugs, so that you can start practicing "root cause" medicine and play a part in solving the epidemic of modern, chronic disease that is destroying our quality of life.

There's no doubt that this is the future of medicine. Cleveland Clinic has seen it, which is why they opened a center for Functional Medicine that already has a six-month wait list for new patients. And millions of people around the world have already reversed chronic diseases ranging from irritable bowel syndrome (IBS) to rheumatoid arthritis with an ancestral diet and lifestyle (which I'll explain in detail later in the book).

My question for *you* is, will you be part of it? Will you join me in this movement to revolutionize healthcare and give people who've been without hope or relief a chance to recover and live their dreams? Will you be ready when a patient like Leo comes into your office?

I hope the answer is a resounding "yes."

FROM BAND-AIDS TO TRUE HEALING

Imagine an approach to healthcare that:

- Prevents and reverses chronic disease, instead of just managing it.
- Offers inspiring, meaningful, and rewarding work to doctors and other practitioners.
- Uses health coaches, nutritionists, and other allied providers to support patients in making lasting diet, lifestyle, and behavior changes.
- Reduces the cost of healthcare for governments, organizations, and individuals.

This might sound like a pipe dream, given how far our

current system is from this ideal. But the good news is clinicians are already seeing success applying this approach in private clinics, primary care groups, and even large institutions like Cleveland Clinic.

This book serves as both a manifesto and a call to action. Chronic disease is a slow-motion plague that is sabotaging our health, destroying our quality of life, shortening our lifespan, bankrupting our governments, and threatening the health of future generations.

If you're reading this book, the failure of conventional medicine to address chronic disease probably isn't a news flash. You wouldn't have bought it if you thought our current system was doing a fantastic job. The problems I'm describing are not secrets; in fact, they're frequently discussed in the media, and among politicians, healthcare professionals, and the public.

But most people don't realize two crucial points. The first is the sheer scale and urgency of the crisis we're facing. As I will argue in Chapter Four, we've reached an inflection point where we can no longer afford *not* to act on a massive scale. The second is that the action we take must not come out of the same system that caused—and continues to cause—these problems in the first place.

As the saying goes, "Insanity is doing the same thing over and over and expecting a different result." We desperately need a *new* approach to healthcare that can address the challenges we face, and an army of healthcare providers—from licensed clinicians to nurses to health coaches to nutritionists—to embrace this approach and start healing the world.

My sincerest hope is that, after reading this book, you'll be inspired to join the thousands of other clinicians and patients who are working together to save humanity from the scourge of chronic disease and usher in this more humane and effective approach to healthcare.

How I Got Here

I've come to this purpose of ending chronic disease through not only a decade of working directly with patients but also as a patient who struggled for many years with chronic disease. In my mid-twenties, I contracted a serious illness while traveling in Indonesia. The acute tropical illness was awful, bringing on fever, chills, vomiting, and severe diarrhea. Far more difficult for me, though, was negotiating the long road to successful treatment of the post-infectious syndrome that lingered long after the first symptoms subsided. Conventional medicine knew how to treat my immediate problems—parasites and dysentery—but when chronic illness set in, nobody knew how to help me. I was exhausted and listless and suffered nearly constant digestive problems, muscle pain, and severe insomnia. I've since recovered from that illness, but the experience changed my life.

I tried everything to figure out what was going on and get help. When I returned home, I went first to my local doctor. Making little progress there, I turned to doctors around the country and then the world. I probably saw thirty different doctors over the course of my exploration. Most had little idea what would fix my problems, so they turned to palliative interventions. Doctors offered medications that would theoretically help with symptoms. Antibiotics initially worked, but left me feeling worse. Some recommended drugs unrelated to my condition, like antidepressants. The suggested remedies were designed to treat my symptoms, but they didn't even do that successfully. Or if they did, they caused other symptoms that were just as bad or worse. Eventually, the doctors would just throw up their hands; they had nothing left to offer. It was becoming clear to me that conventional medicine was not set up to handle the kind of problems I was dealing with.

I tried everything else I could think of. In addition to antibiotics, steroids, and anti-inflammatories, I took hundreds of different supplements and visited experts of all sorts, from psychotherapists to shamans. None of these healing modalities cured me.

Then one day, while browsing in a bookstore, I came across a book called *Nourishing Traditions* by Sally Fallon. Fallon advocated a real-food, nutrient-dense approach to nutrition based on the diets of traditional cultures around the world. (I'll be referring to this later in the book as an "ancestral" diet.) The idea of following a more traditional diet resonated deeply with me, so I decided to give it a shot. I started eating the foods the book recommended, including bone broth, slow-cooked meats, fermented foods, eggs, and cold-water, fatty fish. I eliminated all processed and refined foods, and even whole grains and legumes because I found they didn't agree with me. I felt better almost immediately.

Not long after this, I had my first appointment with an acupuncturist. The acupuncture treatments were the only intervention I had tried, aside from the ancestral diet, that made a positive impact. But what truly impressed me was the way the clinician looked at the whole picture of my health. None of my other doctors had looked at my case from a holistic perspective, but she spent time with me, using a systems approach to try to figure out causes, instead of playing Whack-A-Mole with my symptoms.

As I gathered knowledge, made connections, and continued to heal, people began coming to me with their own questions, and I started informally helping others in their healing processes. I realized that I wasn't alone in my suffering, and that many people were not well-served by the conventional medical system. My own journey had shown me that there must be a better way—not just for me but for others. So I returned to school to study acupuncture and integrative medicine. I was drawn to these modalities; they had helped me make the most progress with my illness.

Shortly after I started school, I attended a seminar on Functional Medicine. I was immediately hooked. I realized that this was the approach to medicine that I had been looking for, both as a patient and as a practitioner in training. It focused on addressing the root cause of disease, instead of just using drugs that work like Band-Aids but seldom fix the underlying problem. I continued to train in Functional Medicine while I finished my acupuncture and integrative medicine degree. By the time I graduated, I knew that Functional Medicine (rather than a traditional acupuncture practice) was my path, and I started a Functional Medicine practice right out of school.

The patients I attracted to my practice were, perhaps not surprisingly, people with experiences like mine: they had chronic, complex, multi-systems illnesses that were poorly understood and even more poorly treated by conventional medicine. They had already seen several doctors, tried numerous treatments, and been told that little could be done for them. They were at the end of the line.

I was grateful for my background in Functional Medicine and an ancestral diet and lifestyle, because these approaches enabled me to help these patients in a way that the conventional system could not. It was amazing to watch chronic diseases of all types—digestive issues, autoimmune diseases, mood and behavioral problems, metabolic disorders, and more—improve significantly and even completely resolve. I became convinced that the combination of Functional Medicine and the ancestral approach was the most effective and powerful means of reversing chronic disease available.

After several years of practicing this way, however, it became clear that something was still missing. I realized that the episodic model of care, where the patient sees a clinician once every three to six months, was simply not sufficient for most patients struggling with chronic disease. They needed more support than I could provide in an occasional thirty-minute appointment, especially when much of that appointment was spent interpreting lab test results and prescribing treatment based on those results.

What if the patient needed more guidance and support on diet, managing stress, adopting a new physical activity routine, or making other important behavior or lifestyle changes? I simply didn't have enough time to provide the level of support in these areas that the patient needed to be successful. I knew that the "expert model" of simply telling the patient what to do, and expecting her to follow through, wasn't enough. (We'll find out why later in the book.)

The answer to this challenge was a new, collaborative model of care that uses allied providers—both licensed clinicians like nurse practitioners and physician assistants, and non-licensed practitioners like nutritionists and health coaches—to provide a much-needed additional layer of support for patients. These allied providers hold the patient's hand through every step of the process, including answering questions about how to complete the lab testing, providing recipes and meal plans, offering guidance on starting a meditation practice or a new exercise routine, or simply providing moral support.

This was like the final piece of a puzzle clicking into place. I had already witnessed the power of Functional Medicine coupled with an ancestral diet and lifestyle, but adding a care model that offered the support patients need to successfully implement the interventions that a functional, ancestral approach prescribes was truly a game-changer.

The Birth of the ADAPT Framework

In 2014, I began to write and speak about a new model of healthcare combining the three elements I've mentioned above—Functional Medicine, an ancestral perspective, and a collaborative practice model—which I call the ADAPT Framework.

ADAPT has multiple meanings. Naturally, it implies adaptation. Our genetic code is hard-wired for a specific environment. When that environment changes faster than our genes can evolve, a mismatch occurs. As we'll see later in the book, this mismatch is the primary driver of the chronic disease epidemic.

The term also suggests that medicine itself needs to adapt. At the turn of the twentieth century, acute, infectious diseases were the top three causes of death, and our medical paradigm evolved in that context. Today, seven of the top ten causes of death are chronic disease. Our system of medicine needs to adapt to better match the challenge of chronic, rather than acute, disease.

Finally, our model for delivering care needs to adapt. Statistics indicate that both practitioners and patients are dissatisfied with the current model. Clinicians are spending less time with patients, finding less meaning and fulfillment in their work, drowning in bureaucracy and inefficient systems, unable to practice the way they want, and not finding what they had originally sought in the practice of medicine. And they are working harder than ever before, without making more money. Patients are not getting the care, support, or answers they seek. They're prescribed drugs that aren't effective (and sometimes cause harm), and little investigation is done to determine the underlying cause of their problems. Therefore, we need to adapt our healthcare model to better serve patients and create a more fulfilling and rewarding career for clinicians.

In 2016, I launched a program to train clinicians in the ADAPT Framework. Since then, we've worked with over 400 clinicians and expect to train more in upcoming sessions. My training program educates a small subset of practitioners, but many more people need to learn about this new model. I hope this book will serve that purpose.

Who Is This Book For?

I'm writing this book for three primary audiences.

Practitioners working in the conventional system

The first audience is MDs, DOs, NPs, PAs, and other practitioners (including students training in these professions) working in the conventional system. This book is for you if you:

- Feel burned out and drained by the "assembly line" style of medicine prevalent in primary care settings today.
- Are tired of ten- to fifteen-minute appointments and managing symptoms with drugs, and want to offer deeper healing and transformation to your patients.
- Want to restore meaning and purpose to your work and rediscover your original passion for medicine.
- Have realized that diet, lifestyle, and behavior are the primary drivers of chronic disease, but feel unable to offer patients adequate support in these areas (or feel that the conventional recommendations are outdated and ineffective).
- Want to have more rewarding relationships with fewer patients, work fewer hours, and have a better quality of life—all without sacrificing income.

This group may also include podiatrists, nurses, registered dietitians, physical therapists, occupational therapists, medical assistants, and even dentists (we have several in our ADAPT training program). There are too many professional titles to list here, but I'm referring to any medical provider working within the conventional system.

Practitioners working outside of the conventional system

The second audience for this book is the wide variety of licensed and non-licensed practitioners (and students training in these programs) working outside of the conventional system. This includes naturopaths, acupuncturists, chiropractors, psychologists, nutritionists, physical trainers, and health coaches—among many others. This book is for you if you:

- Want to upgrade your clinical skills to get better results with patients/clients.
- Are seeking a more comprehensive and systematic framework to apply to patient/client care.
- Have learned about Functional Medicine or the ancestral diet and lifestyle and want to incorporate them into the work you're already doing.
- Would like to form collaborative and mutually supportive partnerships with MDs, DOs, and other practitioners working in Functional Medicine, to better support your patients/clients.

This second audience is a huge group. I believe you will play an increasingly important role in healthcare. As we'll discuss in Chapter Five, there simply aren't enough doctors to address the chronic disease epidemic. Even if there were, most of them have neither the time nor training to support patients in the crucial diet, lifestyle, and behavior changes required for preventing and reversing disease. That's where you come in!

Patients and the public

Finally, this book is for patients who are struggling with a chronic health issue and "citizen scientists and health enthusiasts"—members of the public who are taking their health into their own hands, and are passionate advocates for reinventing healthcare and reversing chronic disease. This book is for you if you:

- Are trying to address a chronic disease or health problem, but do not feel well-served by the care that you're currently getting.
- Have learned about Functional Medicine and/or the ancestral diet and lifestyle, and are seeking a practitioner who uses these approaches.
- Want to help a friend, colleague, family member, or other person you're close with who is suffering from a chronic disease.
- Feel passionate about reinventing healthcare, reversing chronic disease, and optimizing human potential, and want to support this movement however you can.

Although this book is primarily written for healthcare

practitioners, it's also intended for the growing audience of patients and members of the public who question the status quo. Instead of blindly following "expert" advice, you're listening to a variety of voices. You read books and blogs, listen to podcasts, attend summits and conferences, and take in all that you can about how to get and stay healthy. Every time I speak at a conference, several of you approach me to express your passion for this mission of ending chronic disease. This book is for you, too.

CHAPTER THREE

IF NOT NOW, WHEN? IF NOT YOU, WHO?

The writing is on the wall. Chronic disease has devastated our healthcare system, and neither practitioners, patients, nor society at large can escape the effects. If we don't intervene, the situation will only get worse.

Will you answer the call?

There may be a million reasons why you feel now is not the time to take the leap, or why you might not be the right person or in the best position to take this on. I hear you, and I've been there myself.

But there's an old Zen story that has always inspired me in times of uncertainty or self-doubt. One day an old Tenzo (head cook) was washing rice in the temple courtyard in the heat of the mid-day sun. A young monk approached him and asked, "Tenzo, why are you washing rice in this heat? Shouldn't a younger, less experienced monk be doing this kind of work?" The old Tenzo replied, "If not now, when? If not me, who?"

So, given the challenges we face and the dire need for people to join the fight, I'll pose the same question:

If not now, when? If not you, who?

PART TWO

THE PROBLEM

CHAPTER FOUR

CHRONIC DISEASE: A SLOW-MOTION PLAGUE

Conventional medicine has a long record of impressive achievements. Antibiotics revolutionized the treatment of infections from trauma, injuries, and bacterial and parasitic pathogens. Vaccines had a similar impact on reducing the burden of acute, infectious disease. Anesthesia made it possible to perform surgery without the sheer agony and pain that characterized it in the past, and antisepsis (the creation of a sterile surgical environment) greatly improved survival rates after surgical procedures. Radiologic imaging and other laboratory tests and procedures have enabled us to more accurately diagnose disease.

Advances in childbirth (such as anesthesia, cesarean section, and forceps delivery) have significantly reduced infant mortality. Organ transplantation has offered hope for people who would otherwise have no other options.

Collectively, these advances led to a dramatic increase in human lifespan in the industrialized world—especially in the last century. If you were born in 1900, there was a good chance you'd be dead before your fiftieth birthday. Today, if you live in the United States, you can expect to live for seventy-eight years. If you live in other countries like Canada, Japan, or Monaco, your lifespan is even longer: eighty-one, eighty-two, and ninety years respectively.

But these are just averages. Centenarians—people who reach the age of 100 years or more—are the fastest growing segment of the population. Estimates suggest that if the population of centenarians continues to rise at its current pace, there could be close to 1 million people of 100 years of age or more in the United States by the year 2050.

What's more, medical advances have not stopped—they're continuing at an accelerated pace. In our lifetimes, we can expect to see everything from bionic eyes that allow blind people to see, to electronic "defibrillators" implanted in the brain that stop seizures, to precision treatments that kill cancerous cells without harming healthy cells, to robots that can perform certain procedures more safely and effectively than human surgeons.

Sounds incredible, right?

While there's every reason to celebrate these advances, both past and future, it's also important to recognize the other side of this coin: the meteoric increase in chronic disease, and its dramatic effects on our health, our quality of life, and even our lifespan.

A Longer Life, But With Poorer Health

It's wonderful that our lifespans have increased, but if we spend our final years—or even decades—of that longer life suffering from not just one, but multiple chronic diseases, is that something to be proud of? In fact, this is exactly what studies suggest is happening. A paper published by researchers at the University of Southern California found that although lifespans for both men and women increased in the U.S. over the past forty years, so too did the proportion of time spent living with disability and chronic disease. "We could be increasing the length of poor-quality life more than good-quality life," said lead author Eileen Crimmins, USC University Professor and AARP Professor of Gerontology at the USC Davis School of Gerontology (Crimmins et al. 2016).

Imagine a woman, Latisha, who is diagnosed with Crohn's disease at age twenty-seven. She has crippling abdominal pain, indigestion, and urgent diarrhea several times a day. These symptoms make it difficult for her to work, engage in leisure activities, and enjoy her life. She sees a gastroenterologist, and after trying several medications, can at least partially control her symptoms. But the steroid she is taking has significant side effects, including increased appetite and weight gain, particularly around the mid-section. By the time Latisha turns thirty-five, she has become obese and has developed type 2 diabetes. These conditions cause further suffering and require more medication. A few years later, her mother passes away and the stress of that event triggers a flare in her Crohn's symptoms. The medications that had previously controlled it no longer work, so her doctor prescribes infliximab, a biologic drug that is used to treat autoimmune diseases. While infliximab brings her gut symptoms under control again, it causes several side effects, including extreme fatigue, headache, and constant muscle pain. These symptoms interfere with her sleep, and her fatigue worsens.

At some point, the symptoms become so pronounced that Latisha can no longer work. She goes on short-term disability, hoping that she'll be able to recover and return to her job. But after a year, she has not only not improved, she's gotten worse. She didn't have long-term disability insurance, so she goes on Medicaid. Understandably, she becomes depressed. Her physician prescribes an SSRI, which helps to some extent but also causes new symptoms, like dizziness, nausea, and agitation.

By the time Latisha turns sixty-five, she's taking nine prescription medications and several over-the-counter drugs. She is unable to work, has an extremely limited social life, and spends much of her time at doctor's offices and pharmacies, battling with Medicaid representatives to secure care, and researching her conditions. Eventually, Latisha declares bankruptcy because of her growing medical bills. Unable to afford private housing, she is forced to move into a Medicaid-sponsored nursing home, where, against all odds, she manages to live until age eighty-four.

I wish I could say that Latisha's story is unusual; unfortunately, it's all too common. Latisha lived a relatively long life—exceeding the average life expectancy in the United States by several years. But was she able to live a rich and fulfilling life? Were these extra years meaningful and rewarding?

The situation is even more dire with children. The proportion of kids with chronic disease has risen dramatically over the past two decades. Twenty-seven percent of children now suffer from chronic disease, up from just

13 percent in 1994 (Van Cleave et al. 2010). This is heartbreaking. A chronic disease in an adult may mean twenty or thirty years of suffering. But a chronic disease, or multiple chronic diseases, in a child may mean sixty, seventy, or even more years of suffering.

Consider a child, José, who develops asthma, allergies, eczema, and ADHD before the age of ten. And imagine that these conditions persist until he passes away at age eighty-eight. Although these conditions aren't life threatening (except for asthma, which still kills 250,000 people a year), they can be debilitating and significantly reduce quality of life—especially collectively. This means that José will be suffering unnecessarily for *more than seven decades*.

Is this the kind of life we want to live?

Or, a *Shorter* Life With Poorer Health?

Unfortunately, the situation may be even worse than previously described. Recent studies suggest that today's children are the first generation expected to live shorter lifespans than their parents (Olshansky et al. 2005). This should serve as a wake-up call, since life expectancy has been on an upward trend in the industrialized world (a few temporary dips during pandemics notwithstanding) for as long as we've been measuring it.

This projected decrease in life expectancy has been attributed mostly to the explosion of chronic diseases like obesity and diabetes in children. Obesity and diabetes are associated with significant morbidity and mortality, and are primary risk factors for heart attacks and cancer, which remain the number one and number two causes of death in the U.S., respectively.

The Sneaky Rise of Chronic Disease

It might feel like our situation today snuck up on us. But if we look with 20/20 hindsight, we can see that it happened quickly. As recently as the 1950s and 60s, for example, obesity was rare. Our health has changed so dramatically that many of us alive today can remember those days. If you look at family photographs from fifty or sixty years ago, you may be surprised by how much leaner most people were. That's because you've become used to a population where two of three people are overweight and one in three is obese.

Chronic disease is now a defining feature of Western society, and unfortunately, it's also one of our exports. As developing countries adopt our lifestyle and dietary habits, they are also starting to develop these diseases at an alarming rate.

In the next chapter, we'll discuss three reasons why

chronic disease has exploded across the industrialized world. But first, let's take a closer look at just how prevalent—and frankly, alarming—chronic disease has become.

The Colossal Burden of Chronic Disease

It's hard to overstate just how serious this problem is. If we look at the facts, we'll realize we're on a frightening trajectory.

One in two Americans now has a chronic disease, and **one in four** has multiple chronic diseases. Chronic disease causes seven of ten deaths in the U.S. and accounts for 86 percent of healthcare expenditures (and 99 percent of Medicare dollars!), 91 percent of prescriptions, and 76 percent of physician visits (NCCDPHP 2016; NIEHS 2015, 295; Johns Hopkins University Partnership for Solutions 2000).

1 in 2 Americans have a chronic disease; **1 in 4** have multiple chronic diseases.

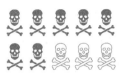

Chronic disease is responsible for **7 out of 10** deaths in the U.S.

91% of all prescriptions filled are for chronic illness.

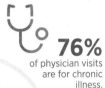

76% of physician visits are for chronic illness.

Chronic Disease

The U.S. spends about

$3.2 trillion on healthcare.

99% of Medicare dollars

86% of that goes to **treatment of chronic illness.**

and **83% of Medicaid** dollars

go to chronic illness.

Spending on chronic disease worldwide will reach

$47 trillion by 2030.

The burden of chronic disease

The financial burden of chronic disease is so enormous it's hard to comprehend. The U.S. spends **$3.2 trillion**

a year on healthcare (Munro 2015). This is equivalent to 18 percent of our gross domestic product, or roughly $10,000 for every man, woman, and child in America. This might not be so bad if these stratospheric expenditures led to superior results. They don't. Although our healthcare system is the most expensive in the world by far, on many measures of performance, it ranks last out of eleven developed countries (Schneider et al. 2017).

The U.S. is certainly worse off than other countries, but that doesn't mean they aren't struggling as well. Chronic disease will generate **$47 trillion** in healthcare costs globally by 2030 if the epidemic is unchecked (Duff-Brown 2017). That's more than the annual GDP of the six largest economies in the world!

Are We Headed Toward a Future Where *Everyone* Has a Chronic Disease?

I wish I could tell you that things are looking up, but that's simply not true. There's every indication that the chronic disease epidemic will get worse before it gets better (unless we embrace the approach I'm advocating in this book, of course).

A new report from the Centers for Disease Control (CDC) found that 100 million Americans—nearly one in three—

have either prediabetes or diabetes (CDC 2017b). A full 88 percent of people with prediabetes don't know that they have it, which is significant because statistics show that prediabetes progresses to full-fledged type 2 diabetes in just five years if untreated. Most disturbingly, the rate of type 2 diabetes in children and teens is increasing by almost 5 percent a year (NIH 2017).

According to the American Autoimmune Related Diseases Association (AARDA), 50 million Americans (approximately one in six) have an autoimmune disease. In comparison, cancer affects 9 million Americans and heart disease 22 million. Researchers have identified 80–100 autoimmune diseases and suspect at least forty additional diseases of having an autoimmune basis (AARDA 2017).

More than 5 million Americans are living with Alzheimer's today, but that number is expected to more than triple by 2050. Every sixty-six seconds, someone in the U.S. develops the disease. Alzheimer's is now the sixth leading cause of death in the U.S.; the number of deaths has increased by 89 percent since 2000. Alzheimer's kills more people than prostate and breast cancer combined, but it doesn't just affect the people who are diagnosed: 35 percent of caregivers for people with Alzheimer's or dementia report that their health has gotten worse due to their responsibilities (Alzheimer's Association 2017).

A recent study documented a 52 percent decline in sperm concentration and a 59 percent decline in total sperm count in men over a nearly forty-year period ending in 2011 (Levine et al. 2017). A decline in sperm count and concentration leads to a decreased probability of conception. The authors of the study speculated that increased exposure to endocrine disrupting chemicals in the environment may be partly to blame for this trend.

Finally, according to the latest estimates, one in forty-five children now have autism spectrum disorder, up from just one in 500 in 1999 (Zablotsky et al. 2015). This is not only due to increased rates of detection. More children will be diagnosed with autism this year than AIDS, diabetes, and cancer combined. The effects of autism are debilitating, far-reaching, and lifelong.

A Slow-Motion Plague

These statistics are unequivocal proof that our current approach to healthcare is failing, and that the consequences are severe. But we don't tend to see this as an emergency as we might if there were a bird flu or pandemic; we just see it as our life.

A better way of understanding the impact of chronic disease is as a slow-motion plague. Although it may not match the scale of the bubonic plague in the Middle Ages in terms of mortality, it's arguably an even bigger problem because of the sheer numbers of people affected and the wide range of those effects. I don't think it's an exaggeration to suggest that our very survival as a species is at stake.

Given this, it's imperative that we embrace a new model of healthcare with the potential to not only stop the increase in chronic disease but reverse it. In the next chapter, I'll explain why conventional medicine, at least in its current configuration, will *never* be able to achieve this goal.

CHAPTER FIVE

THREE REASONS U.S. HEALTHCARE IS DESTINED TO FAIL

It's no secret that our healthcare system is in trouble: countless books, media articles, and scientific studies have explored its many shortcomings in detail. They include:

- **Misaligned incentives.** In the U.S., we rely on insurance companies to pay for care. However, the goals of insurance companies are not always aligned with patient needs, nor with doctors' needs. Insurance companies profit when healthcare expenditures grow. Because of this, there's little motivation for insurance companies to embrace treatments that would ultimately shrink spending on health care. And there's little incentive for doctors, hospitals, or other providers to prioritize quality, efficiency, and cost-effectiveness in their approach.

- **Big Pharma influence.** Like insurance companies, pharmaceutical companies wield enormous influence in the medical industry and are usually motivated by factors other than optimizing care. The incentives to promote a pharmaceutical company's work and products may be more focused on making money than aligning with patient and doctor needs.

- **Bias in medical research.** Two-thirds of medical research is sponsored by pharmaceutical companies, and conflicts of interest, groupthink, and a failure to replicate many findings undermine the credibility of the studies that form the edifice of our current medical paradigm.

- **Broken payment models.** Because we rely on insurance companies to pay for care, the treatments offered are not necessarily the most effective or those supported by the most current evidence—they're simply the treatments that insurance companies have agreed to reimburse. This is not evidence-based medicine, it's *reimbursement-based medicine.*

These problems are real, and collectively they've brought our current system to its knees. But if you've been following the healthcare debate in the news, you might have the impression that if we just make some minor changes here and there, we can get ourselves out of this mess.

That impression is hopelessly misguided.

Making a few small tweaks to our current system and expecting that to work is like rearranging the deck furniture on the Titanic as it inexorably sinks into the ocean. Too little, too late. Why? Because as significant as the problems I've described are, there are three much deeper reasons that healthcare in the U.S. (and in many other parts of the world) is doomed to fail:

1. Our modern diet and lifestyle are out of alignment with our genes and biology.
2. Our medical paradigm is not well-suited to tackle chronic disease.
3. Our model for delivering care doesn't support the interventions that would have the biggest impact on preventing and reversing chronic disease.

Let's take a closer look at each of these reasons.

#1: Mismatch Between Our Genes and Environment

The evolutionary biologist Theodosius Dobzhansky once said, "Nothing in biology makes sense, except in the light of evolution."

What does this mean? All living organisms—including human beings—evolved in a specific environment. Our genes and our biology adapted over tens of thousands of generations to allow us to survive and thrive in that environment. But if that environment changes faster than our genes can adapt, mismatch occurs.

Before farms and factories took over, human beings lived most of our history eating a hunter-gatherer diet and living a hunter-gatherer lifestyle. Our ancestors would hardly recognize modern agriculture and manufacturing or the foods they produce. Our genes have not been able to fully adjust to these changes. The result: a discrepancy between our ancestral genes and the modern environment, which has spurred the chronic disease epidemic.

If you visualize the timeline of human history as a football field, you'll see how quickly our environment has changed. A walk across most of that field—ninety-nine-and-a-half yards out of 100—represents the amount of time we lived as hunter-gatherers. The last half-yard represents the time since agriculture was developed. The Industrial Revolution came along only in the last few inches.

We think the way we live now is normal because it's all we know. It may be all our parents and, to a lesser extent, our grandparents knew. Yet, it's not normal. It's far outside the norm of human evolution and history.

Diet

For most of evolutionary history, humans ate primarily meat and fish, wild fruits and vegetables, nuts and seeds, and some starchy plants and tubers. Nobody ate processed food. Nothing came in a bag or a box. There was no refined sugar, no refined flour, and no industrial seed oil. The only food available was nutrient-dense and whole. Preparation was minimal.

Contrast that with today. The top six foods in the American diet are grain-based desserts, bread, sugar-sweetened beverages, pizza, alcohol, and chicken—primarily fried dishes like chicken nuggets (DIAG 2010). If you put pictures of these two diets next to each other, you'd see a profound difference. We went from a diet that was naturally anti-inflammatory, high in nutrients, and low in calories, to one that is pro-inflammatory, low in nutrients, and high in calories.

Little influences our health more than the foods we consume. The modern diet is a prescription for obesity, metabolic problems, and all kinds of other chronic diseases.

Lifestyle

The mismatch between our evolutionary history and our modern environment goes beyond diet. Consider our exposure to light. If you think about the evolution of humans—indeed, all organisms—you'll see that life evolved in the natural twenty-four-hour light-dark cycle on this planet. We've long used candles and fire to light up the night, but only in the past 100 years have we had the capacity to be exposed to bright, artificial light at times when the sun wasn't shining.

While there's no doubt artificial lighting has been a boon from a cultural perspective—it lets us stay up late to create art, literature, and music, for example—it has had a disastrous effect on our health. We take advantage of expanded daytime to do more activities at night, but doing so disrupts our circadian rhythm. Every cell in our body is regulated by the natural light-dark cycle. When we change that cycle, our bodies suffer.

Here's how it works: When we wake up in the morning, sunlight hits our eyeballs and our cortisol levels rise, telling us it's time to get up. When the sun sets and darkness falls, on the other hand, our melatonin levels rise, telling us it's time to go to sleep.

What happens when someone lies in bed at night with their iPad before going to sleep? The iPad emits blue light, which is like the spectrum of sunlight. When blue light hits the body, it sends a "time to wake-up" message. That not only interferes with sleep but has been shown to deregulate metabolism, promote weight gain, and cause cancer (Chepesiuk 2009). Changes to the circadian rhythm mediated by light exposure can have profound effects on health.

Flight personnel, for example, have long been known to have higher risk of cancer and other diseases, probably due to the circadian disruptions that come from flying across time zones and working at odd hours. By being awake when they should be asleep and asleep when they should be awake, they have upset their body's healthy rhythms. The same happens with people who work night or alternating shifts: they have higher rates of obesity, diabetes, metabolic problems, and cancer (Blask et al. 2009).

Artificial light seems like a benign environmental change, but when you understand it through an evolutionary framework, you begin to see its problems. Then, when you look at the research, you find that yes, in fact, this difference between our ancestral and current environments is significantly harming our health.

One of the most valuable aspects of the evolutionary framework is that it helps us ask questions about our environment we might not otherwise ask. Light is a good example. If we understand that our environment has changed faster than our genes can adapt, we can look at our modern environment and identify the ways it differs from the historic one. We can then investigate and study these differences to see if they have caused problems. If we find they have, this exploration can give us ideas on how to make changes.

For instance, people might decide not to use electronic devices in bed before sleep. They might avoid shift work, or at least advocate for regular, rather than alternating, shifts. They could plan to get some exposure to bright sunlight in the morning before work. Just a week of camping, for instance, can reset the circadian rhythm (Wright et al. 2013). Thinking about it this way reveals a whole realm of possibilities, not just in terms of diagnosing a problem, but solving it.

Behavior

We've known for a long time that exercise is important. That's not a news flash. What might be more surprising is the recent research indicating that going to the gym isn't an adequate solution. If we look at exercise from an evolutionary perspective, we see that our ancestors moved all the time. They walked an average of 10,000 steps a day (Cordain and Friel 2005). They didn't sit for long periods and they stood more than half the day. In between, they chased prey, ran from predators, and built things.

This non-exercise physical activity may be more important than the regimented workouts we're familiar with today. If you work at a desk but go to the gym three or four times a week, you'll meet the conventional guidelines for exercise, but you'll still be at increased risk of disease because of all that sitting. Even marathon runners in training who spend most of the rest of their time sitting have an increased risk of death and disease (Möhlenkamp et al. 2008).

People who walk or are active doing gardening, chores, or manual labor in addition to exercise have a much brighter outlook than those who just exercise. If someone is inactive, it's more important for them to reduce the amount of time they're sitting than it is for them to start a workout routine. The important change for them is to move from being completely sedentary to increasing their non-exercise physical activity.

Why do we continue the behaviors that are obviously causing us so much trouble? Our behavioral patterns are hard-wired for a specific environment. That environment has changed, but our behavioral patterns have not. For example, we're programmed to seek out calorie-dense, highly rewarding foods. Eating potato chips is rewarding: it makes us want to eat more. Eating a plain baked potato will satisfy hunger, but it's not as rewarding.

We're wired to seek rewarding foods because in the past obtaining them would have given us an advantage. These foods have a lot of calories; they prevent us from starving. Starvation was historically the problem for humans, not obesity. Our brains are programmed to help us survive in an environment of food scarcity. Our cravings and desires are set up for that kind of environment.

For instance, there's a hunter-gatherer population in Paraguay, the Aché, that illustrates how strong this programming is. Certain people in the tribe climb extremely high trees, risking their lives, and getting stung by hundreds of bees, just to get honey. When they do get it, people will consume up to a liter of honey at a time. They have no concept of what's healthy or not healthy. They're acting purely out of their evolutionary programming when it comes to food. If you're living in a situation where food scarcity is a problem, it makes sense to use every calorie-dense source of food you can.

What happens when there's a 7-Eleven on every corner selling Big Gulps and jumbo bags of potato chips? We still eat it all, as if it were scarce. Yet we live in a food-abundant environment today. The same behavioral patterns that helped us survive in a natural environment now make it very likely we're going to become overweight and develop metabolic problems and other chronic diseases.

The mismatch between our evolutionary inheritance and our modern environment lies at the root of chronic disease. This mismatch is causing a massive health crisis in America and the West that our current health systems are ill-equipped to manage.

To address this, we need to adopt diet and lifestyle behaviors that are species-appropriate, acknowledging the ways humans have evolved to survive in an environment very different from the one we live in today. If our current diet and lifestyle are totally at odds with our natural history, we must make different choices to bring ourselves back into alignment. Choosing a diet that is more closely aligned with our genome and epigenome acknowledges that, although our ancestral diet varied according to what was available, there were some common characteristics: There was no processed food. People ate some combination of meat, fish, wild fruit and vegetables, nuts and seeds, and starchy plants, no matter where they lived. They weren't eating Ding Dongs, Cheez Doodles, and Big Gulps.

We'll discuss how to realign our diet, behavior, and lifestyle with our genes in more detail in Chapter Nine.

#2: The Wrong Medical Paradigm for Chronic Disease

Our current medical paradigm is based more on managing disease and suppressing symptoms than it is on preventing and reversing disease, or promoting health.

Conventional medicine is structured to address trauma, acute infection, and end-of-life care, not to keep people healthy. Imagine a linear spectrum, where death sits on the far right and perfect health on the far left. Conventional medicine intervenes at the right end of the spectrum. The closer a patient gets to death, the less chance a clinician has of restoring that patient to health. Yet, that's precisely where we spend our greatest resources. Heroic interventions can prevent death, but don't necessarily promote health.

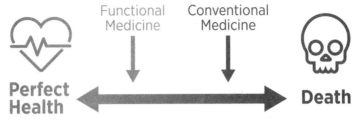

Functional Medicine | Conventional Medicine

Perfect Health ⟵⟶ Death

The spectrum of chronic disease

Don't get me wrong: modern medicine is incredibly effective in acute and trauma care. If I get hit by a bus, I want to be taken to a hospital! Fantastic advances in medicine have turned what was previously limited to the realm of science fiction into reality: we can restore sight to the blind, re-attach limbs, and even clone human stem cells. We absolutely need oncology surgeons who can remove cancerous tumors and gastroenterologists who know how to perform a colonoscopy. But I think we can all agree that conventional medicine does not excel at preventing or reversing chronic disease, which is the biggest challenge we face today.

One reason for this is that there has been a fundamental change in the healthcare landscape throughout the past century. Our healthcare paradigm evolved during a time when the top three causes of death were all acute, infectious diseases: typhoid, tuberculosis, and pneumonia. In 1900, you might have visited a doctor for an accident or injury, a gallbladder attack or appendicitis, or an infection—not because you had an autoimmune condition, allergies, or asthma.

1900	2016
Typhoid	Cardiovascular disease
Tuberculosis	Cancer
Pneumonia	Lung disease

Top causes of death in the U.S., by year

Treatment for these issues was relatively simple: the doctor removes the gallbladder or appendix, sets the broken bone in a cast, or gives the patient medicine for an infection. One problem, one doctor, one treatment.

Early in the twentieth century, antibiotics revolutionized the treatment of infections. Previously unimaginable cures became common. If a patient had an infection, she took an antibiotic and shortly thereafter was cured. Cause and effect seemed clear. The "one disease, one treatment" mentality was applied to other medical procedures as well, such as surgery.

Surgery seemed efficient—if the appendix was going to burst, surgical removal would fix the problem in one fell swoop—and was widely celebrated. Surgeons made amazing discoveries and began saving lives with their new techniques. People who once had no hope could now survive, if they had access to the right surgeon. Surgeons were treated like gods.

Today, the healthcare landscape has changed dramatically.

Seven of the top ten causes of death are chronic diseases (NCCDPHP 2016). Unlike acute problems, chronic diseases are difficult to manage, expensive to treat, and usually last a lifetime. They don't lend themselves to the "one problem, one doctor, one treatment" model that worked well in the past. **Today's patient has multiple problems, sees multiple doctors, and requires multiple treatments that go on for years if not decades.**

Another reason that conventional medicine hasn't been successful is that it focuses on suppressing symptoms rather than addressing the underlying cause of disease. Imagine you get a rock stuck in your shoe, and it makes your foot hurt. If you look for help in the current medical system, you may get a description of foot discomfort along with directions to the nearest drugstore for some extra-strength ibuprofen. Sure, ibuprofen would help to reduce the pain. But wouldn't it be better just to take off your shoe and dump out the rock?

For example, patients regularly arrive in doctors' offices with myriad health issues related to diet, such as obesity and/or diabetes. After meeting with a doctor, they'll walk out with prescriptions for insulin and drugs that lower blood sugar. While these drugs might be crucial to maintaining a diabetic's health, they won't ultimately solve the patient's chronic disease. A Type II diabetic requires a lifestyle change: patients need to remove unhealthy processed foods and refined sugars from their diet. Most doctors know and advise this, but our current medical system doesn't support patients to make the lifestyle changes required for long-term solutions. The result? Patients continue to live with chronic disease, and doctors continue to prescribe them medication for symptom management.

But perhaps we're not being fair. In the examples listed above, it's likely that a skilled conventional medical practitioner *would* identify the rock in the shoe. It's possible that a persuasive doctor would adequately convince a patient to initiate a lifestyle change, and conceivable that a motivated patient would go home and diligently apply those changes. That is, of course, if the issue is as simple as identifying just one rock.

In most cases, there's more than one rock. The first pebble might be a patient's poor diet. The next comes from sleep deprivation, a result of going to bed at 3:00 a.m. and only getting five hours of sleep at night. Another rock is born from sitting at a desk for eight hours a day and failing to do any exercise. A patient who has accumulated several rocks like this needs medical advice that considers the whole picture, not merely the acute presenting symptoms.

Some rocks are nearly invisible. Perhaps a patient, Yolanda, is dealing with a disease like irritable bowel syndrome (IBS). Typically, Yolanda would go to the doctor and leave with a handful of medications, all of which simply suppress symptoms without addressing the cause of her problem. Yet, there are often mechanisms or pathologies at work that require further exploration. Yolanda might have something called SIBO, or small intestinal bacterial overgrowth, which involves inappropriate growth of bacteria in the small intestine. Maybe she has an undiagnosed food intolerance, or an undetected parasite infection. She might have a gut-brain axis problem caused by an autonomic nervous system issue, like sleep loss or stress. An array of mechanisms may be driving the condition, and, unfortunately, they often remain undiscovered—or at least go unaddressed.

In a ten-minute appointment, there simply isn't time to thoroughly investigate all the possible causes of a patient's chronic illness. Instead, doctors describe the symptoms and prescribe the drugs, and that's the treatment. If that doesn't solve the issue, the patient usually gets referred to a specialist, who, as we've seen, examines one area of the body in isolation. If the chronic issue persists, the patient is sent to another specialist, who examines another area of the body, and then another specialist, *ad nauseum*. Unfortunately, it's rare for those specialists to communicate with one another; our current medical system isn't set up to accommodate that kind of collaboration. Primary care doctors are supposed to unify the various discoveries, but their overwhelming caseloads often make it impossible.

What would it be like, instead, if doctors were empowered to approach illness like a detective approaches a case? After considering the patient's host of symptoms, this doctor asks, "What might be causing those symptoms? Let's do some thorough testing to determine what some of the causes might be. Once we identify those causes, we'll start removing them and see if you still have those problems. We won't rule out using drugs if necessary, but we're going to focus our energy on identifying the root causes of your symptoms and addressing them all." This is how Functional Medicine operates.

We'll talk more about Functional Medicine in Chapter Eight.

#3: A Healthcare Model That Doesn't Support Preventing and Reversing Disease

"The wise physician treats disease before it occurs," according to the Traditional Medicine proverb from the Huangdi Neijing, an ancient medical text. Unfortunately, there's simply no framework for that in current practice. The interventions we need to address the chronic disease epidemic require investing our resources in promoting health, which is just the opposite of what we are doing today.

At one time, it seemed that genetics would hold the key to solving chronic disease. Recent studies, however, have found that **84 percent** of the risk of chronic disease is not genetic, but environmental and behavioral (Rappaport 2016). Our genes do play a role in determining which diseases we're predisposed to developing, but the choices we make about diet, physical activity, sleep, stress management, and other lifestyle factors are far more important determinants of our health.

It's tempting to think that we can solve this problem simply by better educating people about the changes they need to make. But lack of information is not the issue. Most people know that eating poorly, not exercising, not getting enough sleep, and engaging in other unhealthy lifestyle habits is not good for them. Yet they continue these behaviors anyway, or they chase quick fixes that don't last for more than a few weeks.

What about doctors? Shouldn't they be the ones to lead this change? We simply don't have enough of them to address the problem. The most recent statistics suggest that we'll have a shortage of 52,000 primary care physicians by the year 2025 (Petterson et al. 2012). But even if we didn't have a shortage of doctors, most of them have neither the training nor the time necessary to support people in making lasting behavioral changes. We could start training doctors and other healthcare providers in this area, but that still wouldn't solve the problem. Our "sickcare" system is not set up to deliver this type of care.

The average visit with a primary care provider (PCP) in the U.S. lasts for just **ten to twelve minutes** (Yawn et al. 2003), with newer doctors spending as little as eight minutes with patients (Chen 2013). It is *impossible* to deliver high-quality care in eight to twelve minutes when a patient has multiple chronic health problems, is taking several medications, and presents with new symptoms. Such brief appointments leave little to no time to dig into the important diet, lifestyle, and behavioral issues that are causing the patient's symptoms. And with an average of 2,500 patients per provider, it's difficult for PCPs to develop the kind of relationship with patients that would support meaningful changes.

Even if a provider makes a suggestion about diet or lifestyle change, will it be successful? It is now widely accepted that knowledge is not enough to change behavior. Yet doctors are trained in the "expert model" of simply telling people what to do, and expecting them to do it. That might work well when someone is facing a serious, acute health crisis (like an appendicitis), but it fails miserably when it comes to long-term behavior changes like losing weight, managing stress, or adopting an exercise routine (Elfhaq and Rossner 2005). Doctors aren't trained to work collaboratively with their patients. This is painfully reflected by the fact that patients get to speak for only twelve seconds on average before being interrupted with advice from their physician (Rhoades et al. 2001).

If we continue to schedule short appointments with doctors, we also need to arrange lengthier visits with health coaches or other allied providers who can work more intensively with patients.

Imagine the healthcare population as a pyramid. The top 5 percent of the pyramid—those experiencing acute or emergency problems that require intensive care, often in a hospital or specialized outpatient setting—are often best served by conventional medical intervention. They need the kind of acute intervention conventional medicine excels at.

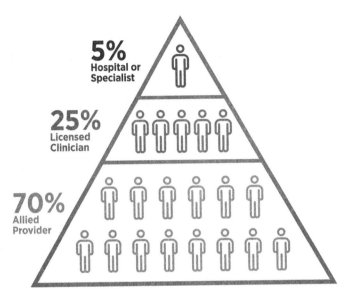

5%
Hospital or
Specialist

25%
Licensed
Clinician

70%
Allied
Provider

The Healthcare Population Pyramid

The next 25 percent of patients in the middle of the pyramid—those dealing with significant chronic health challenges—will likely require the ongoing support of licensed clinicians practicing Functional Medicine (with or without a conventional physician, depending on the scope of practice of the Functional Medicine provider and the specific health challenge).

The 70 percent of patients at the foundation of the healthcare pyramid—those with less severe chronic health problems—can often be adequately served by allied providers (such as nurse practitioners or physician assistants, nutritionists, and health coaches) focusing on diet, lifestyle, and behavior change, with occasional visits to a licensed Functional Medicine clinician. These people could join those at the higher levels of the pyramid at any time if they don't address their diet and lifestyle, which is exactly what happens in today's conventional medical paradigm.

We'll talk more about a new practice model that better supports key interventions for preventing and reversing chronic disease in Chapter Ten.

CHAPTER SIX

THE TOLL: HOW CONVENTIONAL MEDICINE AFFECTS HEALTHCARE PROVIDERS

A growing number of practitioners who started in conventional medicine are making their way to a Functional Medicine approach. Why? To put it plainly, the conventional system leaves them feeling burned out.

A recent survey we did at Kresser Institute revealed the impact of the conventional system on practitioners.

We asked our students whether the statements below described them "totally," described them "well," described them "somewhat," and so on. Here's what they said:

- "I am disillusioned with conventional medicine."
  - 40 percent answered, "This describes me totally."
  - 42 percent answered, "This describes me well."
  - 16 percent answered, "This describes me somewhat."
  - 2 percent answered, "This doesn't describe me."
- 37 percent said they feel inspired by their work.
- 25 percent said that when they wake up in the morning they look forward to their day.
- 73 percent said they're dedicated to their patient's well-being.
- 59 percent frequently feel overwhelmed in terms of having too much to do in the time available to them.
- 39 percent said they feel overwhelmed by paperwork.

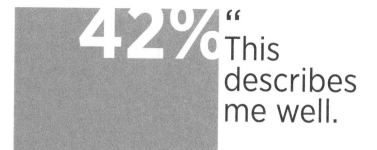

42% " This describes me well.

40% " This describes me totally.

16% " This describes me somewhat.

2% " This doesn't describe me.

Percentage of clinicians disillusioned with conventional medicine (Kresser Institute, 2017)

These responses describe a group of people who long to care for their patients well. Yet, they're being worn down by a system that makes it extremely difficult to provide that care. Functional Medicine, with its longer appointment times and smaller patient loads, can help the 75 percent of survey respondents who don't wake up looking forward to their day. If they know they can have more meaningful relationships with patients, support from allied providers, and access to high-quality diagnostic tests, the workday looks a lot brighter. They can finally make the difference they want to make in patients' lives and health.

What does this look like? In this chapter, we'll explore some real stories of clinicians who became dissatisfied with conventional medical practice, and found the fulfillment of their calling in Functional Medicine.

Insufficient Time Leads to Deficient Quality

Both doctors and patients feel dissatisfied with how little time gets spent on doctor-patient visits. This enables doctors to see more patients per day—often around twenty-five or more—but at the expense of in-depth care. A typical primary care physician (PCP) has a total of 2,500 patients on their roster. A more reasonable number of patients for optimal quality of care would be closer to 1,000 or even 500 (Schimpff 2015, 5). In other words, a typical primary care doctor is being pushed to treat up to five times the number of patients as is recommended for best practice. The focus has been on quantity when doctors should be focused on quality.

Financial Pressure

Unfortunately for physicians, this increase in appointments has not been met with an increase in income. After inflation-adjusted terms, primary care doctors earn somewhat less today than they did in 1970, yet they see twice the number of patients. Most medical school graduates have large debt: the average amount is $170,000, while 40 percent of medical school grads owe more than $200,000 (Schimpff 2015, 8). Even though it's widely agreed upon that doctors earn a decent income, their high levels of debt fuel the reimbursement environment. Doctors are paid per patient, which is part of what drives the high patient load. Given the high levels of debt most doctors enter medicine with today, a PCP must see twenty-five or so patients a day to earn $170,000 to $220,000 a year—the amount needed to keep paying off $200,000 of debt. Although many doctors might wish for a smaller patient load to increase quality of care, the financial reality makes that challenging to maintain.

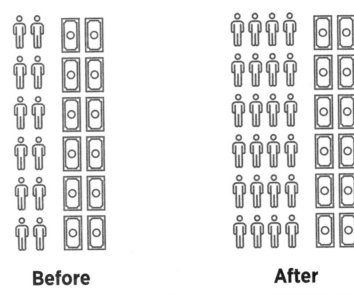

Before **After**

Patient care in 2014 vs. 1970: working harder, but earning less (Schimpff 2015, XIX)

Professional Dissatisfaction

It's no wonder physicians suffer from burnout. They fear that their efforts are failing to have the positive impact they envisioned when they first got into medicine. The statistics listed below (The Physician's Foundation 2016) are telling:

- 63 percent of physicians are pessimistic about the future of the medical profession.
- Half of physicians "often" or "always" experience feelings of burnout.
- 54 percent of physicians rate their morale as "somewhat" or "very" negative.

- Only 14 percent of physicians have the time they need to provide the highest standards of care.
- Almost half of physicians are thinking of quitting medicine, cutting back hours, switching to concierge medicine, or taking other steps to limit patient access.

63%

of physicians are pessimistic about the future of the medical profession.

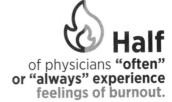

Half

of physicians **"often"** or **"always" experience** feelings of burnout.

Side Effects of Practicing Medicine

54%

of physicians rate their morale as **"somewhat"** or **"very" negative.**

Only
14%

of physicians have the time they need to **provide the highest standards of care.**

Almost Half

of physicians are thinking of **quitting medicine, cutting back hours, switching to concierge medicine,** or taking other steps to **limit patient access.**

The "side effects" of practicing medicine (The Physician's Foundation 2016)

Clearly, doctors are feeling unhappy. After a long day of seeing twenty-five patients, many doctors feel like they haven't been able to help all, or even many, of the patients they've seen. That's a prescription for serious professional dissatisfaction. Stephen Schimpff writes in *Fixing the Primary Care Crisis*, "Many PCPs feel like they're on the clock. Instead of maintaining a professional attitude, they're beginning to act like...a Home Depot mentality. Instead of high quality, the concept is to see how many patients they can fit in during one day." In the words of Sherry, a practitioner we'll hear more from later in this chapter, it's "factory medicine."

The long hours typically served by doctors only add to this professional dissatisfaction. Typically, a PCP might have thirty to forty hours of patient care on their weekly calendar. Sounds reasonable, right? Not when you consider that means sixty to seventy total hours in the office, plus on-call hours. The constant work schedule leaves little time for research or new learning; other life-giving practices, like self-care or time with family, are pushed to the sidelines. Burnout seems inevitable.

Unfortunately, the problem is likely to grow worse. Estimates indicate that America currently has approximately 210,000 primary care physicians in an active practice but will need an additional 53,000 by 2025 (Petterson et al. 2012). This estimate assumes that each PCP will see 2,500 patients each. If we accept the premise that PCPs should be seeing 500 to 1,000, there will clearly be many more physicians needed.

People drawn to the medical profession are not afraid of hard work, but hard work that doesn't seem to do a lot of good leads to profound professional disillusionment. As the stories in this chapter reveal, many medical practitioners are hungry for a better way—and many have found it through shifting to a Functional Medicine model.

A Better Way

What's the antidote to burnout? Imagine seeing a patient make meaningful changes and get better from the inside out as they start addressing the root causes of their problems. Or watching a patient leave from an appointment feeling hopeful for the first time in memory. Imagine working with a long-suffering patient who had endured all kinds of complex and risky procedures, multiple diagnostic tests, and years' worth of visits to a clinic without seeing results. Might a doctor feel reinvigorated after helping this patient feel better after she applies a simple recommendation related to diet or supplements?

That's certainly how I felt when I treated Mary, a senior vice president at a tech company in Silicon Valley. Over the last several years, she'd noticed a steady decline in cognitive function. It started with what she described as brain fog, an inability to concentrate as well as she was accustomed to. Over time, this progressed to poor memory and even worse brain fog. It got to the point where, by the afternoon, Mary felt unable to do her job. She also had become short of breath, particularly when she exercised, and was less tolerant of exercise. Workouts she had no problem with just a couple years before seemed impossible now. She was having a lot of digestive issues, including constipation, gas and bloating, pain, and some reflux.

Mary went to top doctors in San Francisco and Silicon Valley, and some just told her she was getting older and the symptoms were simply part of aging. Others said they were all stress related, and diagnosed her with depression and anxiety, even though she wasn't depressed and didn't particularly feel anxious. She underwent sophisticated testing and procedures to rule out Alzheimer's and dementia, and ended up being prescribed several different medications: antidepressants, Ritalin for attention, sleeping pills, and medications for the digestive symptoms. None of them helped in a significant way. She was concerned about the side effects and being stuck taking these drugs for the rest of her life, especially when they weren't particularly helpful.

When Mary came to see me, I ran some simple, but complete blood work and noticed that her serum B12 level was low-normal. Not out of the lab range, but below optimal and at a level that has been associated with B12 deficient symptoms in the scientific literature. Homocysteine and another marker called methylmalonic acid were high (these are inverse markers of B12 deficiency, which means if they're high it suggests that B12 is low). I also determined that Mary had small intestinal bacterial overgrowth (SIBO), which is associated with a deficiency of B12 and many other nutrients (Dukowicz et al. 2007). When you put all this together, it was suggestive of B12 deficiency.

For Mary, discovering these underlying causes was a game-changer. I suggested adding some animal products to her mostly vegetarian diet, particularly shellfish and organ meats which are extremely dense in B12. We treated her SIBO so she could absorb the B12 better, and we started her on a sublingual B12 supplement to get her levels up quickly.

The change was dramatic and almost immediate. She said it felt like someone had turned the lights back on after she'd been living in the dark for a very long time. In fact, in one follow-up appointment she got emotional. She said, "I might have gone my whole life this way thinking this was just part of aging. Who knows, I might have eventually been diagnosed with dementia or even Alzheimer's when it was really just B12 deficiency and correcting it was as simple as taking a vitamin and changing my diet."

I've heard other patients say something similar. It's a tremendous relief when you find the underlying cause of a problem and you're able to address it relatively simply, and it's often a life-changing experience because it brings with it a flash of insight into what the future might have been without this discovery.

These are the kinds of moments that abound when practicing Functional Medicine, and moments like these are when the work starts to get fun. Clinicians start saying things like, "I can't imagine retiring," or "I can't imagine ever getting bored." When once burned-out medical practitioners can look forward to a lifetime of learning, they feel hopeful and energized in a way that they haven't in recent memory. It's impossible to state the value of waking up and feeling excited about the day, with the knowledge that your work will make a difference in people's lives. Practitioners of Functional Medicine have control over their practice methods. They determine how they structure appointments with patients and even how they interact with those patients. That's priceless.

Clinician Stories

Let's look at a few more stories from clinicians who have made the transition from conventional medicine to Functional Medicine and the ADAPT Framework.

Sherry

Sherry went to medical school imagining her future practice would look something like a Norman Rockwell painting. She assumed she'd get to know her patients, spend time with them, and help them get better. The reality was shockingly different. She was appalled, for instance, at how her colleagues in government healthcare treated diabetes. From very early on, she realized that her dietitian colleagues were recommending a conventional dietary paradigm to their diabetic patients: a low-fat, high carbohydrate diet. Even high-glycemic products were considered okay, if patients stuck to the carb count set forth for them. She attended internal medicine conferences sponsored by some of the major-name distributors of what many would consider junk food. Soda and donuts filled the food tables at these conferences. Sherry was floored.

Sherry advised her diabetic patients to stop eating bread, but the dietitian she worked with scolded her in response. Bread was a key component of the low-fat diet they were prescribing! She remembered receiving only a brief lecture on vitamins in medical school and had no nutritional training whatsoever, but she knew from her personal life as an athlete that this advice had to be wrong. Suspecting that nutrition played a pivotal role in her patients' chances of recovery, she picked up *The Blood Sugar Solution* by Mark Hyman, MD, one of the pioneers of Functional Medicine. That book introduced her to Functional Medicine, and she immediately recognized its value.

Sherry had heard of integrative medicine, but had mostly ignored it. In her mind, it lacked a cohesive framework and wasn't evidence based. However, when she learned that Functional Medicine sought to understand a patient's root cause for illness, she saw that it was grounded in systems biology and immediately knew it was right for her.

Her experience left her feeling like a cog in a patient mill—like she had been practicing factory medicine. She saw a seemingly endless number of patients, but at the end of the day, Sherry still felt like she hadn't helped anybody. The hours passed in a nonstop blur of writing on her prescription pad and offering pills to patients. Some days, she didn't even have time to go to the bathroom. As a result, she felt increasingly frustrated and depressed—a prescription for clinician burnout. But when she found Functional Medicine, she felt like she had finally found her passion.

After switching to a Functional Medicine approach, Sherry began to see significant changes in both her methods as a physician, and her patients' experience with her. One of the biggest modifications in her practice was how she approached autoimmune disease, which is now epidemic. Conventional medicine falls woefully short in addressing the complex nature of autoimmune disease; often the solutions offered consist of little more than steroids or painkillers—nothing that addresses root causes. With Functional Medicine, Sherry can significantly improve the lives of her patients. She has been able to get her patients off medications entirely, and help them feel better. Word spread as friends and family members saw the results Sherry was getting with her patients. They started contacting her and pleading for appointments.

Eventually, Sherry started a small private practice so she could help these people. The time slots she had filled up quickly. As Sherry approaches retirement, she's working toward establishing a full-time Functional Medicine practice. This is not only more appealing professionally, but will also be a better fit for her lifestyle. The collaborative approach that I advocate in the ADAPT Framework means that Sherry will eventually be able to have a more flexible work arrangement—something highly prized by a mom of six kids. Right now, she has to live close to work to see her patients at the hospital. But once she has a full-time Functional Medicine practice, she imagines a more distributed, virtual setup. When she's in her home town, she can see some patients in person, and she can also do telemedicine video consultation. Consulting remotely would enable her to travel to visit her kids, while still maintaining her practice.

When Sherry was practicing conventional medicine, she was counting down until retirement. Now, she doesn't see herself retiring at all. She has found her Functional Medicine practice to be both fulfilling and liberating in its flexibility. Most important of all, Sherry experiences enormous joy in helping people—truly helping people— who are sick become well.

Caroline

A psychiatrist who worked for twelve years in a conventional setting, Caroline was a community doctor in an outreach clinic. She enjoyed her residency in psychiatry, and went on to treat many patients with serious mental illnesses like schizophrenia and depression. As a psychiatrist, Caroline recognized the role of the mind in a patient's overall health; psychiatry acknowledges some connections other specialties don't. Caroline's initial training in psychotherapy encouraged her to think holistically about patient health. Even so, she always had a nagging feeling that something was missing from psychiatry.

Some of Caroline's patients took five to six psychiatric medications. The possibility of drug interactions alarmed her. One afternoon, Caroline was sitting out in her garden—a beautiful, dense area where she often retreated to be in nature. As she sat there, she had an epiphany: she realized that if a patient of hers died because of the dangerous interaction of their various psychiatric medications, she could never sit peacefully on that bench again. This powerful realization made her determined to move to a more holistic, integrative approach. This is when she moved into private practice.

So, she tried. She began incorporating supplements, nutrition, and herbs, working to get people off medications. However, her approach felt haphazard. Ultimately, she was still functioning within the conventional paradigm; she was using supplements and herbs to deal with symptoms, instead of using a root cause approach. Her practice still felt like it was missing something. Then, like Sherry, Caroline read a Mark Hyman book: *The Ultra Mind Solution*, published in 2009. Before she was even halfway through Hyman's book, she was on the Internet reviewing Institute for Functional Medicine (IFM) training, Functional Medicine, and clinical practice. She became passionate about Functional Medicine. Caroline describes it as an incredible adventure: "I feel like I'll never be bored for the rest of my life," she has said.

The biggest difference between treating patients before and after Functional Medicine? "Before, most of my patients had no hope," says Caroline. "The diagnosis was depression or anxiety and the treatment was drugs. When I was asked how long they would have to take those drugs, the answer was, 'for the rest of your life.' It was understood that those drugs were not correcting anything permanently. So, the patients often felt hopeless." Caroline also points out the irony that apathy itself is a side effect of many of these drugs. When working under a conventional medicine paradigm, a patient who says they're depressed and apathetic receives an increased dose of drugs, perpetuating a vicious cycle. Caroline often looked through clients' files and saw a lengthy trail of medications they'd already taken and found ineffective or harmful. At that point, she wondered what she had to offer them.

That doesn't happen to Caroline anymore. Now that she uses a Functional Medicine paradigm, her patients leave feeling hopeful—sometimes they even feel better by the end of the first appointment. That has dramatically changed the mood of her meetings, and creates a much more positive experience working as a practitioner. Now, Caroline feels she has a tremendous array of tools to offer. The results that she gets with her patients have been radically transformed, and because of this, her work with the patients has been transformed as well. She's excited and passionate in a way that she never was with conventional medicine.

Andrea

When Andrea was six, her two-year-old sister was diagnosed with leukemia. Andrea spent most of her childhood in and out of hospitals visiting her sister, until her sister finally passed away when Andrea was ten years old.

Although her family didn't find naturopathy until after her sister had passed, Andrea went to a naturopath as her primary care doctor after that. The naturopath quickly resolved Andrea's mononucleosis infection and helped her mother avoid a hysterectomy. The naturopath's approach was interesting to Andrea, even at a young age. She was fascinated by how the body worked and by medicine in general. Even at ten years old, she sensed that something about the way medicine was being practiced wasn't quite right. Doctor's appointments lacked warmth and feeling, even though Andrea felt like those qualities were important parts of helping someone get better. Not surprisingly,

Andrea pursued a pre-med path in college. Still, something about the field of study didn't resonate with her.

Although Andrea tried a few other pursuits like real estate and starting her own business, she kept feeling pulled back to medicine. She valued the holistic approach to medicine she'd seen when her family had visited the naturopath, but she also felt it was important to get more knowledge in the conventional approach. As she had ruled out being a doctor, she decided that becoming a nurse practitioner was a good compromise.

When she graduated from nursing school, Andrea initially set her sights on emergency medicine. Even after years of study, she still didn't feel like she had the tools she needed to truly care for and nurture people. Although she had learned diagnosis codes, acquired a prescription pad, and possessed a big heart and an interest in helping people, she suspected that wouldn't be enough to help people in a meaningful way.

From the beginning, Andrea had hoped to find a way to bring the Eastern and Western perspectives on medicine together, feeling like either approach on its own was incomplete. The Western approach of conventional medicine felt devoid of warmth and feeling, as she'd discovered with her sister. It also failed to consider health problems holistically and seemed to ignore important aspects like nutrition. But the alternative medicine approach also seemed flawed. Some of the alternative medicine modalities seemed haphazard and not sufficiently systematic. Too often practitioners would just use supplements and herbs to treat symptoms, rather than truly shifting to root cause medicine. She wanted something that had the systematic approach of Western medicine, and the holistic paradigm of Eastern medicine.

Finally, Andrea found what she was looking for. Throughout her professional and educational journey, Andrea had never heard of Functional Medicine—but that changed when she was online one day. An ad for Institute for Functional Medicine (IFM) popped up. Andrea was intrigued. She took the Applying Functional Medicine in Clinical Practice course, and although she gleaned some great information, she yet again felt a desire for more practical systematization. How could she apply the paradigm? Then she discovered the ADAPT Practitioner Training Program and her goals for practicing medicine all came together. The ADAPT training was practical, provided a systemized approach, and offered a community of other people with whom she could interact and exchange ideas.

Throughout her journey toward Functional Medicine, Andrea had been seeing patients at a free clinic in Oakland,

California. Many of those patients were under significant socioeconomic stress, with symptoms related to digestive issues, fatigue, or insomnia. They were distressed and feeling poorly, but since they didn't have a clearly defined disease like diabetes or cardiovascular disease, they were often written off as "fine" by the doctors there. At times, patients were prescribed an antidepressant or similar medication, but not given again any meaningful route to feel better.

Andrea recognized early on that some of these patients needed a different solution. In one case, she saw a woman who complained of gut issues, fatigue, and insomnia. The woman was also under significant stress. In a long effort to resolve her medical problems, this woman had endured a colonoscopy and an endoscopy; she'd taken a host of medications, and had been coming to that clinic for three years, seeing multiple doctors and practitioners. After all of that, she didn't feel like she was making any progress. Andrea took a simpler approach with the woman. She recommended that the patient try taking digestive enzymes which could be found cheaply on Amazon, and gave the woman some dietary recommendations. Something as simple as a digestive enzyme and the changes in diet enabled the woman to finally turn a corner with her health. Experiences like these confirmed Andrea's belief that a Functional Medicine approach was the best way to help her patients in a meaningful way.

Amy

Amy trained as a radiologist and did a fellowship at Stanford in Pediatric Radiology. Amy's patient list included kids at eight or nine years old with morbid obesity, diabetes, and autoimmune conditions. Some even showed blood markers of inflammation and fatty liver. Radiologists don't typically see patients directly. They consult more with doctors and discuss the interpretation of scans. Even though Amy wasn't often interacting directly with the kids, she would notice many of them sitting in the waiting room eating Cheetos or drinking a big soda, focusing exclusively on their iPads. Despite the obvious need for lifestyle changes, there was no discussion of nutrition, diet, or exercise in what she observed between the primary care physician, the team of specialists, or their parents. This struck Amy as producing a clear disconnect in achieving proper care for the pediatric patients.

Around that same time, Amy started experiencing a decline in her health. She was getting closer to her mid-thirties, and experiencing a range of bothersome symptoms: trouble sleeping and energy crashes, trouble with her weight for the first time in her life, and irregular cycles. She went to see an OB/GYN, where she waited two hours for a fifteen-minute appointment. During the visit, few labs were ordered and she was quickly diagnosed with Polycystic Ovary Syndrome (PCOS) solely based on her symptoms. She was prescribed metformin, a blood sugar medication typically prescribed to diabetics, even though she had normal blood sugar. As a physician and radiologist, Amy was a skilled researcher—and this didn't add up to her. She looked up PCOS and saw that she clearly didn't meet the criteria for that diagnosis. Two weeks later, the diagnosis changed: she was told she had hypothyroidism and was prescribed thyroid hormone. The medical conclusions handed to Amy seemed overly hasty. She felt as though no one had taken the time to thoughtfully consider what was going on in her body, and no one, including herself, stopped to consider how her work schedule with nights on call allowing for little more than a few hours of sleep, while training for a half Ironman triathlon, might play a role in her health and well-being.

Around that period, Amy read *Good Calories, Bad Calories* by Gary Taubes, which questions the mainstream dietary dogma. Following that, she researched the Paleo diet, which led her to my work, blog, and book. She was immediately drawn to this approach to health and well-being. She had seen enough working with pediatric patients and her own health that it just made sense. Still, Amy initially felt reluctant to fully pursue Functional Medicine. She'd made a huge investment in the conventional paradigm; after attending years of medical school, she had completed five years of residency and fellowship training at Stanford. These experiences maintained a hold on her, despite her suspicion that there might be a better way. Amy's disillusionment with conventional medicine progressed as more of a slow, steady unraveling, than a rapid paradigm shift. Eventually Amy decided to go in the direction she recognized as the best fit for herself and how she saw best to help others heal, and made the change to Functional Medicine.

For Amy, the biggest benefit of the shift she's made has been finding a career that allows more meaning and satisfaction. As she looks back on her career journey, she realizes now that she chose Radiology for some of the wrong reasons. She enjoys connecting directly with patients and asking them whether they're living in alignment with who they are. She's able to have the kind of in-depth conversations that she could never have when she was a radiologist. Now, she feels better able to make meaningful changes in patients' lives and help them to transform from the inside out.

Christian

When Christian was asked why he entered medicine, he said, "Because my dad expected me to." He is the son of a first-generation doctor who grew up in abject poverty in Montreal, Canada. Out of this poverty, his father had been tremendously successful as a physician, and Christian's dad wanted the same experience for his son. He expected Christian to achieve highly and become a professional of some kind—attorney, physician, architect, or something as equally impressive. As a young man, Christian was ready to comply with his father's vision for his life. After growing up in Canada, Christian went to medical school in Ireland, then came to the United States. Initially, Christian leaned toward pursuing surgery, but when he got to the United States and saw what was expected from surgeons in terms of workload and hours, he panicked and thought, "No way."

During Christian's medical internship, he observed that the only specialty doctors he ever saw with any leisure time at all were the anesthesiologists. This lifestyle seemed far more appealing to him than the surgeon's schedule! Christian went on to achieve the kind of career success that would make his father proud. He became the section head of pediatric cardiac anesthesiology at Cleveland Clinic. Though he'd found success as an anesthesiologist, Christian faced personal disappointments and a rough patch in his marriage. This heartbreaking turn of events caused a major awakening in Christian, and he was forced to re-evaluate what was important to him. He went on to engage in intensive therapy, which helped him face his demons. He saw what wasn't serving him anymore and what areas of his life he needed to let go. He emerged from therapy a different person, one with new views and new priorities.

At that time, Christian was having some of his own health issues as well. He learned of Mark Sisson's Primal Diet, and adapted his diet accordingly. One day while driving, Christian noticed his brain was clear in a way that it never had been before. He knew he was onto something, despite his own past reservations about alternative medicine. Changing to the Paleo diet had really helped him. Christian had previously assumed that anything outside of conventional medicine was "quackery," integrative medicine and holistic medicine included. Now, he wasn't so sure.

Christian started training with A4M, the American Academy of Anti-Aging. Still, he felt he needed more concrete guidance and practical application, which he found in the ADAPT Practitioner Training Program. That training gave him the confidence to apply to Cleveland Clinic Center for Integrative Medicine, the sister clinic to the Center for Functional Medicine. Christian transitioned from Cleveland Clinic Center for Integrative Medicine to Cleveland Clinic Center for Functional Medicine in 2016, where he currently works two days a week, leaving the other three days open for his work in pediatric cardiac anesthesia.

PART THREE

THE SOLUTION

CHAPTER SEVEN

A NEW MODEL: THE ADAPT FRAMEWORK

The chronic disease epidemic is one of the most significant challenges humanity is facing today. This insidious, slow-motion plague is causing untold suffering for hundreds of millions of people around the world; leaving doctors and other healthcare professionals drained and dispirited, and eroding their faith in medicine; and stealing valuable financial resources from governments, corporations, and individuals.

I wish I could say that the stories I told in Part One about Leo and Latisha were unusual. Unfortunately, my practice is full of such patients—and I know the same is true for healthcare practitioners around the world. Perhaps you're dealing with similar challenges yourself, or maybe you have an aunt, a co-worker, or a child who is. With one in two Americans suffering from chronic disease, and one in four suffering from multiple chronic diseases, not one of us is untouched by this epidemic.

Chronic disease has become our reality, and we tend to just accept it as normal. But as I explained in Chapter Five, there's a big difference between what's common, and what's normal. It's *not* normal for human beings to develop chronic disease—especially as children. It's *not* normal for us to suffer and be in pain for years, much less decades. It's *not* normal for us to have to take a fistful of medications just to function at a sub-par level.

In Chapter Five, I argued that there are three fundamental reasons why our conventional healthcare system has not only failed to address chronic disease but will *never* be able to do so in its current configuration. First, it ignores (or pays lip service to) the mismatch between our genes and our modern environment. Second, our medical paradigm is optimized for treating acute, rather than chronic disease. Third, the way healthcare is delivered doesn't support the most important interventions for preventing and reversing chronic disease.

It follows, then, that the solution to the chronic disease epidemic must address *all three* of these shortcomings. Anything less will fall short. In this section of the book, I will describe a solution that does exactly that: the ADAPT Framework. It consists of three elements:

- **A Functional Medicine** approach, which is focused on preventing and reversing, rather than simply managing, chronic disease.
- **An ancestral diet and lifestyle**, which reflects the recognition that we are evolutionarily mismatched to our environment and that this mismatch is the primary driver of chronic disease.
- **A collaborative practice model**, which offers clinicians a structure that better supports delivering Functional Medicine and ancestral diet, lifestyle, and behavioral interventions to patients.

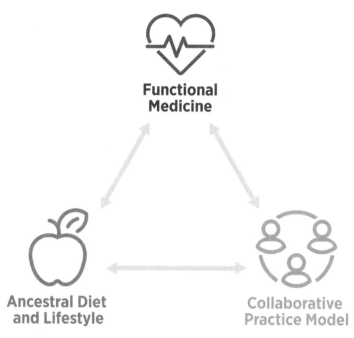

Functional Medicine

Ancestral Diet and Lifestyle

Collaborative Practice Model

The ADAPT Framework

I'll describe each of these elements in detail in the following chapters. But before I do that, I'd like to tell you more about how I developed this framework, and why I believe it's our best option for ending chronic disease.

The Evolution of the ADAPT Framework

I arrived at the ADAPT Framework not only through research and studying larger trends, but through my own experience—both in my personal healing journey, and in my work with patients. You may recall from the introduction that I suffered from a debilitating, chronic illness that took me nearly a decade to recover from. My first big step forward came when I discovered the ancestral health approach. I brought my diet and lifestyle into closer alignment with what my genes and biology are hard-wired for. My second step forward came when I worked with the acupuncturist. Although she wasn't practicing Functional Medicine per se, her approach embraced many elements of it, and it launched me toward learning more. Finally, as I adopted the principles of ancestral health and Functional Medicine, I assembled a team of practitioners that could support me in the various areas I needed help in: a doctor who practiced Functional Medicine, a bodyworker who helped unwind the tension in my gut, a therapist who supported me in addressing the psychological and emotional challenges of my chronic illness, a meditation teacher who continued to guide me in my practice, and several other healers, teachers, coaches, and supporters over the years.

Later, when I started to work with patients, I made the same discoveries all over again. I already knew of the ancestral diet and lifestyle and Functional Medicine from my own healing journey. As I started to use these approaches with patients, I quickly learned that one was not enough without the other.

Functional Medicine provided the crucial shift in focus

from symptom suppression and disease management to preventing and reversing disease by addressing its underlying cause. Yet most Functional Medicine seminars and training programs I attended did not embrace the ancestral diet and lifestyle. Certainly, they advocated for the importance of diet and lifestyle change in general, but the recommendations they made were based more on a plant-based, low-fat diet, which was a disconnect with what I had come to believe from my research, my own healing journey, and my work with patients. The ancestral perspective was important for two reasons. First, it provided an important frame and context for sharing diet and lifestyle recommendations with patients. Second, the recommendations that came out of this frame were far more effective than any other approaches I'd used in the past.

On the other hand, I also learned that the ancestral diet and lifestyle—though extremely effective in most cases—was often not enough to completely reverse the patient's health problems and restore optimal function. Functional Medicine offered a more comprehensive toolset, with cutting-edge laboratory testing and evidence-based treatment protocols using botanicals, supplements, and when necessary, targeted and safe medication.

Finally, as I gained more experience working with patients,

I saw that as powerful as Functional Medicine and the ancestral perspective were, their potential could not be fully realized without a care model that supported these interventions. Consider a patient we'll call Nguyen. She came to see me with a long list of symptoms, including neuropathy, muscle and joint pain, brain fog, memory loss, anxiety, insomnia, constipation, gas, bloating, cold hands and feet, dysmenorrhea and abnormal menstrual cycles, asthma, allergies, frequent ear infections, acne, eczema, dry eyes and mouth, weight gain, and food intolerances.

After a thorough initial work-up, I discovered that she had a parasite (*Giardia*), Hashimoto's thyroiditis, elevated mercury levels, B12 and folate deficiency with borderline anemia, vitamin D deficiency, HPA axis disruption (often erroneously referred to as "adrenal fatigue"), impaired methylation, low estrogen, progesterone, and testosterone, and several other problems. Her treatment involved an antimicrobial protocol to address the gut infections; a thirty-day elimination diet (based on ancestral diet principles); a mercury detox protocol; specific foods and supplements to increase her B12, folate, and vitamin D levels, and improve methylation; and an intensive behavior and lifestyle protocol involving stress reduction, improved sleep hygiene, circadian regulation (reducing her exposure to artificial light at night, and increasing her exposure to sunlight during the day), gentle physical activity, more time outdoors (especially in natural environments), and a meditation practice.

Nguyen clearly needed a Functional Medicine and ancestral diet and lifestyle approach. But let me ask you this: do you think her treatment would be successful with just a thirty-minute appointment with me every three to six months? This is, unfortunately, still the default model even in most Functional Medicine practices. One of my biggest regrets is not realizing the deficiency of this model sooner; I feel sad when I think of the patients like Nguyen who we weren't able to help because we couldn't provide the support they needed.

That's where the collaborative practice model comes in. It provides a methodology and structure for offering patients like Nguyen the tools, resources, and support they require to successfully implement the Functional Medicine and ancestral health protocols. Instead of only seeing a clinician once every three to four months for thirty minutes, Nguyen will have a fifteen-to-thirty-minute check in with a nurse practitioner or physician assistant by phone or video conference every two weeks while she's on her protocol. She can also work intensively with a health coach, who will help her with her new diet (providing recipes, meal plans, and tips for shopping, travel, and eating out) and support her lifestyle and behavior changes. Nguyen may also sign up for one of the groups or classes our clinic might offer for people dealing with specific conditions, such as chronic pain, autoimmune disease, or digestive distress. Through the patient portal in our electronic health record (EHR), she has access to her labs, a library of handouts with guidance on her protocols, appointment scheduling, and a messaging system where she can communicate with her practitioners.

This is a night-and-day difference from her experience with her conventional doctor, where she had less than fifteen minutes to describe her symptoms, no investigation was done to discover their root cause, and the only treatments offered were drugs that either didn't work or caused side effects that were worse than her original complaints. But it's also a significant difference even from most Functional Medicine clinics, where the episodic model of care—periodic appointments with the licensed clinician, with little support offered in between—is still common. Nguyen's experience is exactly why this third element of the ADAPT Framework is so important.

Ready to learn more? Let's dive in.

CHAPTER EIGHT

THE PARADIGM SHIFT: FUNCTIONAL MEDICINE AS TRUE HEALTHCARE

Imagine you're in a boat, and the boat is leaking. You can bail water from the boat to make it sink more slowly, but if the leaks are still there, you'll have limited success. Conventional medicine is mostly about trying to bail water out of the boat without fixing the leaks. Wouldn't it make more sense to prevent the leaks from happening in the first place, and then fix them completely if they do occur? We might still need to bail some water initially, but if the leaks get fixed, the boat is steadied. Eventually, there's no more bailing required, and the sailing—or living—can resume. That's what Functional Medicine is all about.

Root Cause

Functional Medicine seeks to get to the bottom of things. It looks for the underlying cause of disease. Conventional medicine, on the other hand, is organized primarily around suppressing symptoms with drugs and surgery. What does this split look like to a patient?

Say Dorothy goes to a conventional medical doctor with high cholesterol and is prescribed a medication to lower it. It's unlikely anyone investigates further to find out why her numbers are high in the first place, or to help Dorothy make sense of these complex factors. The doctor may mention diet and lifestyle changes, but the system is simply not set up to support these changes.

The Functional Medicine Systems Model

How do Functional Medicine practitioners identify the root cause? I visualize the determinants of health as a series of concentric rings, which I call the Functional Medicine Systems Model.

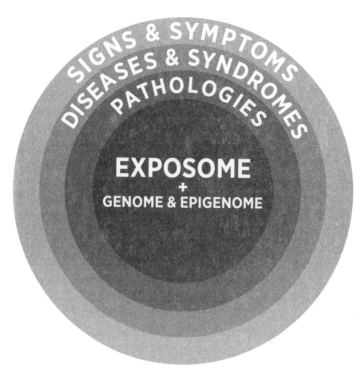

SIGNS & SYMPTOMS
DISEASES & SYNDROMES
PATHOLOGIES

EXPOSOME
+
GENOME & EPIGENOME

The Functional Medicine Systems Model

The Exposome, Genome & Epigenome

At the core of the model is the relationship between the Exposome, our genes themselves, and the way our genes express themselves over time. The Exposome is the sum of all non-genetic exposures an individual encounters from the moment of their conception to the moment of their death. It's a new word that encompasses all aspects of our behavior and environment, including our diet, lifestyle, air and water quality, toxins, social environment, family system, and so on. We know that most diseases are driven by factors related to the Exposome, but the way that disease manifests in an individual is determined by the relationship between those factors, their genes, and their genes' expression. The Functional Medicine Systems Model holds that any progress in a patient's health must start here at the core.

Pathologies

The next ring out from that central core is pathologies. When our modern diet, lifestyle, and environment changes the expressions of our genes, it can lead to deviations from normal physiology that characterize and constitute diseases and syndromes. In other words, pathologies are the underlying mechanisms that *give rise* to diseases and syndromes.

Let's consider a syndrome like IBS. Genetic predisposition combines with environmental influences (such as poor diet, stress, sleep deprivation, exposure to toxins, etc.), which in turn affect gene expression. These interactions lead to pathological mechanisms—such as gut infections, parasites or bacterial infections, low stomach acid, bacterial overgrowth in the small intestine, or a disrupted gut microbiome—that can cause the syndrome that we call IBS. Pathologies also are found in the formulation of many diseases. Insulin resistance and inflammation are two of the pathologies that give rise to type 2 diabetes. Nutrient deficiency and autoimmunity are often at the root of hypothyroidism.

At the core of the Functional Medicine Systems Model lies the relationship between the Exposome, genes, and genetic expression; the next ring out concerns the pathologies that rise out of that core relationship. The ring beyond that depicts the syndromes and diseases that stem from pathologies.

Diseases and Syndromes

What, exactly, is a disease? What's a syndrome?

A disease is defined as a disorder of structure and function that produces specific signs and symptoms. Some examples of diseases are type 2 diabetes, gastroesophageal reflux disease (GERD), Alzheimer's disease, celiac disease, and rheumatoid arthritis.

A syndrome is a group of signs and symptoms that consistently occur together, or a condition characterized by a set of associated symptoms. Some common examples of syndromes are IBS, restless leg syndrome, chronic fatigue syndrome, fibromyalgia syndrome, or premenstrual syndrome (PMS).

A disease is more clearly defined and characterized than a syndrome because it has specific signs and symptoms and the causes are more clearly defined and understood.

Signs and Symptoms

From syndromes and diseases, the circle stretches out to "signs and symptoms." A sign is an *objective* indication of a disease or syndrome that can be observed during a physical examination or through laboratory testing. Examples of signs include the high blood pressure, high blood sugar, and lower leg edema that a physician might observe in a patient with type 2 diabetes. Symptoms, on the other hand, are the *subjective* experiences that the patient might report to the clinician. For the type 2 diabetes patient, symptoms might include increased hunger and thirst, blurred vision, and fatigue.

The signs and symptoms ring describes the outward manifestation of everything that comes before it within the circle. It tends to be the most visible, since the symptoms are generally the way that patients experience what's happening deeper within their body, and the signs are what the clinician observes by examining and testing the patient.

Returning to Dorothy, our earlier example, if a doctor measures Dorothy's cholesterol and tells her, "You have high cholesterol," the doctor is describing a sign. In conventional medicine, they more often see this as a disease itself. In the functional model, we view it as a manifestation of a pathology that results from the interaction between the patient's genome, epigenome, and Exposome. If Dorothy is eating a diet that interacts badly with her genes, that will lead to a pathology—in this case, that might be the improper clearance of cholesterol-carrying lipoproteins from the blood. Eventually, this leads to high cholesterol, the manifesting sign of the other factors at work.

An even simpler example is migraines. If a patient reports having migraine headaches, he's clearly describing a symptom. Headaches are not a disease; they're not even a pathology. Headaches are a symptom, but the conventional model might address them simply with a prescription for painkillers. This approach might alleviate the current headache but does nothing to help us discover the pathologies that lead to the headaches in the first place.

The conventional model typically seeks to manage disease, slow its progression, and help the patient live with symptoms. In some instances, when diseases aren't curable or reversible, those are the only options a healthcare provider may have available. But most of the time, this is an incomplete approach to patient health. It misses the opportunity to prevent and reverse disease, because it works *from the outside in*, focusing mainly on symptoms.

Inside, Out vs. Outside, In

In Functional Medicine, we approach treatment from the *inside of the circles and move outward.*

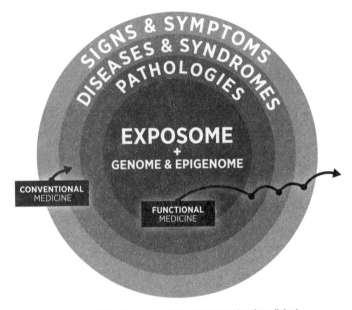

Inside, out (Functional Medicine) vs. outside, in (conventional medicine)

We start with the relationship between the Exposome, the genome, and the epigenome. If we go back to Dorothy's high cholesterol example, the Functional Medicine practitioner might do some testing not only of Dorothy's cholesterol and lipids but also her genetic profile.

For instance, the clinician might determine Dorothy's APOE phenotype. If she is APOE 3/4 or 4/4, or if she has other genetic variants that affect cholesterol and lipo-protein trafficking, the clinician knows Dorothy may be hyper-responsive to the dietary effects of cholesterol and saturated fat. If Dorothy has been trying to lose weight on the Atkins diet, eating few carbs but lots of fat, she may not be doing herself any favors. She might be better off reducing her overall fat intake, and switching out saturated fats for monounsaturated fats. Without the genetic tests, Dorothy may never have realized it.

Consider another patient, Sujata, who comes in with a history of frequent miscarriages. After genetic testing, we might find that Sujata has two copies of a polymorphism in the MTHFR gene. This would predispose her to having low folate levels, and a higher risk of miscarriage. We would recommend that Sujata boost her dietary folate intake—eat more dark, leafy greens, organ meat, lentils, etc. We may also suggest folate supplementation. Once again, we begin with the "inside" and work out, starting with a patient's Exposome.

It's not always necessary (or even possible) to do genetic testing. In many cases, we can use the assumptions of the ancestral model, which recognize that our genes and our biology are hard-wired for the diet and lifestyle that we evolved with for thousands of generations. We can make diet, behavior, and lifestyle choices based on that assumption, when genetic testing isn't available.

After analyzing the Exposome layer, we examine pathology. For Dorothy, several possibilities come to mind. Poor thyroid function, or hypothyroidism, can lead to high levels of LDL particles in the blood. Insulin and leptin resistance also have this effect. If Dorothy is overweight and has diabetes, addressing her insulin and leptin resistance may lead to lower levels of lipoproteins in her blood. We can also consider testing for exposure to toxins—heavy metals like mercury and lead can cause high levels of LDL. In Functional Medicine, we look at all of the potential underlying pathologies, and address them one by one. It's likely that Dorothy would see a reduction in her LDL particle number as she went above and beyond the dietary and lifestyle changes we first suggested.

How Functional and Conventional Medicine Differ

To get a more complete picture of how Functional Medicine works, let's consider it on a broader scale, especially as it compares to conventional medicine. (Note that the comparisons below are generalizations. Just as no two Functional Medicine practices operate the same way, no conventional practices are identical; many clinics and clinicians will fall outside these generalizations.)

Functional Medicine	Conventional Medicine
Optimizes health	Manages disease
Collaborative, patient-centered model	Expert, doctor-centered model
Biochemical individuality	Everyone is treated the same way
Holistic	Specialized
Cost effective	Expensive
Relieves symptoms by addressing cause	Suppresses symptoms with drugs
Preventative approach	Early detection of disease
High touch/High tech	High tech

Comparison of Functional Medicine and conventional medicine

Healthcare vs. Disease Management

As we've discussed, conventional medicine is well-suited for dealing with acute, infectious disease, trauma, and injuries. However, it falters in addressing chronic disease, which is the biggest health problem we face today. This is revealed in the following concerning statistics (Goldhill 2013):

- Within conventional medicine, pharmaceuticals are the primary treatment for almost 90 percent of all chronic conditions.
- At any given moment, roughly 50 percent of American

adults, including nine of ten adults older than sixty, are taking at least one prescription drug.

- Almost a third of adults take two or more drugs.
- Almost 30 percent of all teens are now on a prescription drug, as are 20 percent of young children in the United States.
- America spent just under $310 billion on pharmaceutical drugs during 2015 (IMS Health 2016).

As patients struggle to alleviate their symptoms, they're often given little more than a prescription to solve their problems. The focus of most interactions in conventional medicine is not optimizing health; it's managing disease once it has already occurred. **Conventional medicine is not truly healthcare—it's disease management.**

Functional Medicine, on the other hand, is designed to *promote health.* We try to prevent disease from occurring in the first place, and when it does, we seek to reverse it completely by investigating its underlying cause. You can think of Functional Medicine clinicians as "health detectives."

If a clinician can identify and address the root of problematic symptoms, patients don't just receive a Band-Aid for their problem; they can experience profound and long-lasting results. Conventional medicine, with its emphasis on drugs that are often taken indefinitely, creates "patients for life." Functional Medicine, on the other hand, supports patients to recover their function so they can "graduate" from care and get back to living their life.

Patient-Centered vs. Doctor-Centered

In Functional Medicine, patients are encouraged to play an active and engaged role in their treatment because we recognize that the patient's behavior is one of the biggest, if not *the* biggest, contributor to chronic disease. We believe that if patients want to overcome a chronic ailment, they must shift their behavior.

Our model is patient-centered. In contrast, conventional medicine tends to be doctor-centered, functioning in the "expert" model of care. The doctor provides the answers, and the patient passively receives that expertise.

Of course, not all conventional doctors work this way. Many would never presume to talk down to their patients. Still, the model itself presumes that the doctor is the gate-keeper of information and advice.

Biochemical Individuality vs. En Masse Treatment

We're often asked this question at our clinic: "Do you treat [insert name of disease]?" That's a fair question.

But in Functional Medicine, we don't treat diseases. We treat patients, and the underlying patterns that give rise to disease. We recognize that each patient is unique, and that a one-size-fits-all approach isn't effective. Even patients with the same condition may get different treatments.

Let's say you have two patients—Steve and Miranda—who are each struggling with a skin problem like psoriasis. In Steve's case, we may do some testing and find that he has a gut infection and that's what's driving his condition. We might treat Steve using either antimicrobial herbs or a combination of antibiotics and probiotics. These treatments might resolve Steve's skin condition. But what if we find that Miranda's symptoms stem from an autoimmune disorder? Her treatment will focus more on her diet and supplements to help regulate her immune system, eventually resolving *her* problem. Both patients came to you with psoriasis, but the cause of their symptom—and thus the optimal treatment—is different.

In conventional medicine, two patients with the same condition are likely to receive identical treatment. If Steve and Miranda go to the doctor's office with psoriasis, both patients get the steroid cream, regardless of the underlying cause. The cream may help in both cases, but their skin problems are unlikely to go away completely because the cause hasn't been addressed.

This is one of the reasons why most Functional Medicine practitioners are generalists, rather than specialists. We're less concerned with the specific manifestations (i.e., signs and symptoms) of each disease than we are with the underlying pathologies that give rise to all diseases, signs, and symptoms. The Functional Medicine Systems Model that I introduced earlier in the chapter is the best way I've found of illustrating this distinction, and I often find myself sharing it with both patients and clinicians who I'm training, to clarify the point.

Holistic vs. Specialized

Functional Medicine treats the body as an interconnected whole. It's holistic. We recognize that to treat one part, the other parts must be considered because they're connected.

Conventional medicine, on the other hand, is dualistic, viewing the body as a collection of separate parts. That's why we see specialists for each part of the body, e.g., a cardiologist for heart problems, an endocrinologist for thyroid issues, a rheumatologist for autoimmune conditions. Unfortunately, those specialists infrequently consult with each other or acknowledge the important connections between the body's various parts. It probably wouldn't even occur to Steve's dermatologist to refer him to a gastroenterologist to check for gut dysfunction because, like most conventional medicine specialists, dermatologists don't tend to look at the roots of disease in a systemic fashion.

Cost vs. Savings

One shortcoming of Functional Medicine, at least at the time of this writing, is that it's not well-covered by insurance. This has led to criticism that Functional Medicine is more expensive than conventional medicine. It's true that the accessibility of Functional Medicine is limited because of the lack of insurance coverage, and this is a real problem. But this is largely because conventional medicine is heavily subsidized by the insurance model, whereas Functional Medicine is not. If we examine the actual cost of care—without the insurance subsidies—we'll see that Functional Medicine is often **much more affordable than conventional medicine**, largely because it seeks to prevent and reverse disease, rather than just manage it.

Let's take type 2 diabetes as an example. The American Diabetes Association estimates that it costs approximately $14,000 a year to care for each patient with type 2 diabetes. If a patient develops diabetes at age forty, and lives for another forty years, that's a cost of more than **half a million dollars** to treat a single patient through his lifetime.

If we used a Functional Medicine approach, however, we'd do preventative testing with patients that would catch an early problem with blood sugar long before it progressed to diabetes. We might spend more up front on testing, preventative care, diet and lifestyle intervention, and other treatments than in the conventional model—let's say $5,000, for the sake of argument. But although the upfront cost may be higher, Functional Medicine would save an enormous amount of money over this patient's lifetime, because it would prevent diabetes before it occurred in the first place.

The reactive nature of conventional medicine, which often doesn't intervene until a patient's disease has already progressed, results in massive costs. Patients with advanced disease need more appointments, specialists, tests, checkups, medication, and so on. These costs may not be visible to the patient, since his insurance company is footing the bill, but that doesn't mean they're not real—and it doesn't mean the patient isn't paying for them in some form via insurance premiums, taxes, and out-of-pocket expenses.

High Touch

Functional Medicine takes a "high touch" approach. That means we strive to offer a high level of service to patients. We talk with patients, listen to them, learn about their backgrounds, and provide a level of connection and support that we know is therapeutic itself. This used to be the norm. Just fifty years ago, medical doctors still did house calls and spent ample time with each patient. Modern conventional medicine, with its ten- to twelve-minute visits, instead creates a factory-like, impersonal atmosphere. Functional Medicine is trying to reclaim that higher level of service with the patient.

We also embrace the most recent technology, which helps us provide patient services like telemedicine and to function smoothly as a collaborative team. We use "high-tech" to be "high touch." Conventional medicine embraces modern technology as well, but it often creates a barrier between doctor and patient, rather than a connection.

Integrative Approach

Functional Medicine is integrative, combining the best of allopathic and holistic treatments. We typically start our work with diet, lifestyle, and behavior modifications, nutritional supplements, and botanicals. We don't rule out medications or even surgery when necessary, but they're rarely the first methods that we turn to—mainly because in most cases, drugs don't address the underlying problems. Conventional medicine tends to be more allopathic in its approach, and relies almost exclusively on drugs and surgery. Although most doctors acknowledge the importance of diet and lifestyle, the model isn't structured to support patient change in those areas.

Our integrative approach and treatment protocols also tend to be safer. Functional Medicine treatments typically have fewer side effects, risks, and complications than the drugs prescribed in conventional settings. In fact, Functional Medicine sometimes leads to *positive* side effects. For example, our psoriasis patient Steve not only cured his skin problem by healing his gut and changing his diet, but his digestion and energy improved as well.

Treatments in conventional medicine tend to be more dangerous. Drugs and surgery can cause serious side effects and complications, including death. Some drugs have side effects that are worse than the patient's original symptoms. As a result, many people end up on multiple drugs—some for the original problem, and others for the side effects caused by the first drugs. Consider a patient, Sarah, who takes a medication for anxiety. The medication may help Sarah with her anxiety, but it might also cause constipation. Sarah must then take a medication for constipation, but this medication has side effects as well—and so on. Before you know it, people are on five, six, seven, or eight drugs—or even more.

According to a commentary by Dr. Barbara Starfield published in the *Journal of American Medical Association*, medical care is the third leading cause of death in this country (Starfield 2000). But since only 5 to 20 percent of iatrogenic events (i.e., events caused by medical intervention) are reported, Dr. Starfield speculated that medical care may in fact be the leading cause of death. That frightening statistic stems from prescription drug errors, hospital-related errors, and other iatrogenic events. The functional model holds that often most of a patient's healing can be accomplished through much gentler treatment approaches.

THE HISTORY OF FUNCTIONAL MEDICINE

Although recent history has worked against it, holistic medical care is not a modern invention. In fact, it's ancient. Practitioners of traditional Chinese medicine and Ayurveda, for example, have considered patient ailments comprehensively for centuries. These approaches view human beings as whole beings, rather than a collection of separate parts. Functional Medicine, however, offers key updates. We use state-of-the-art diagnostic tools to effectively identify root causes. Today, we have access to tools like blood, stool, urine, and saliva testing—many of the same tools conventional doctors use. Functional Medicine considers the results of those tests within the ancient paradigm, to establish a meaningful context.

Functional Medicine as a modern pursuit was organized, defined, and clarified by Dr. Jeffrey Bland. Jeff Bland is the founder and president of Personalized Lifestyle Medicine Institute. He's a biochemist, with dual degrees in biology and chemistry. He also has a PhD in organic chemistry. He's a fellow of the American College of Nutrition where he's a certified nutrition specialist.

Dr. Bland didn't originate the concepts of Functional Medicine; they're found in many of the systems of traditional medicine. However, he is largely responsible for organizing and articulating the modern Functional Medicine approach, beginning with his founding of Institute for Functional Medicine (IFM) in 1991. IFM started off small, but over time, it became the largest international organization dedicated to the advancement of Functional Medicine as a treatment approach.

If Jeff Bland is the grandfather of Functional Medicine, Dr. Mark Hyman is the father. Dr. Hyman has been arguably more responsible for advancing Functional Medicine than anybody other than Bland. His work has reached a wider audience than anyone else's—Hyman's books have been number one best-sellers on the *New York Times'* list ten times. He could be considered Functional Medicine's most prolific ambassador.

Cleveland Clinic was the first major organization to recognize the power of Functional Medicine. They tapped Mark Hyman to create a Center for Functional Medicine within Cleveland Clinic. Their practice is booming. They've hired a fistful of new doctors, yet still have an eight-month waiting list. Clearly, a lot of people have been waiting for something like Functional Medicine for a long time.

The Functional Approach to Chronic Disease

Let's examine how these two paradigms—one, looking at a body as a collection of parts, and the other, looking at the body holistically—look different in practice.

Physician's Perspective

Alzheimer's Disease

Dr. Dale Bredesen is a well-established and highly respected Alzheimer's doctor, a scientist who spent decades focused on Alzheimer's research, looking through a microscope in a lab, seeing the trees but not the forest. After many years, he realized how limited this approach was. He hadn't answered some of his most persistent questions: Why is Alzheimer's so much more prevalent today than it was before? Why do contemporary hunter-gatherers seem to escape Alzheimer's? What could explain that? We share many of the same genes with hunter-gatherers, so there must be environmental causes—if that's true, what are they? These questions led Dr. Bredesen to switch to a Functional Medicine approach on his own before he had even heard the phrase.

Dr. Bredesen now addresses dementia and Alzheimer's disease from a holistic—functional—perspective. When a patient comes to see him, he doesn't simply administer memory tests. He investigates the patient's gut function.

He measures their blood sugar. He examines their diet and their nutrient status. He considers heavy metal toxicity, mold, and biotoxins. He analyzes methylation. He looks at detoxification.

Dr. Bredesen is so thorough because he understands that the brain is not removed from all other bodily systems. Inflammation in the gut can affect the brain, and high blood sugar can cause insulin resistance. Insulin resistance in turn affects the availability of glucose in the brain, which is why some people call Alzheimer's "type 3 diabetes."

Dr. Bredesen understands that heavy metals and other toxins cause inflammation and affect the brain and cognitive function. He realizes that vitamin B12, choline, and other nutrients are crucial for brain function. He has restructured his Alzheimer's investigations using this functional perspective, and he summarizes this revolutionary approach in his book, *The End of Alzheimer's: The First Program to Prevent and Reverse Cognitive Decline* (Bredesen 2017).

The results of Dr. Bredesen's "root cause" approach to dementia and Alzheimer's disease have been extremely encouraging. In some cases, patients have seen an almost complete reversal of their symptoms and have been able to resume their work and normal activity. This is unheard of in conventional treatment. In fact, despite more than twenty-five years of trials, not a single drug has been developed that has been shown to slow—much less reverse—the progression of Alzheimer's. In other cases, patients may not see a full reversal of their condition, but at least a slowing or stopping of the progression, which is again more than conventional treatment can offer.

Autoimmune Disease

Another example of how the functional and conventional paradigms differ is Dr. Terry Wahls' approach to autoimmune disease. Dr. Wahls is a clinical professor of medicine at the University of Iowa Carver College of Medicine in Iowa City, where she teaches internal medicine residents in their primary care clinics. She also does clinical research and has published over sixty peer-reviewed scientific abstracts, posters, and papers.

In 2000, Dr. Wahls was diagnosed with multiple sclerosis (MS), and by 2003, she had transitioned to progressive secondary MS. She underwent chemotherapy to slow the disease and began using a tilt-recline wheelchair because of weakness in her back muscles. By 2007, she was in a wheelchair, and the prognosis was that she'd eventually become bedridden by the disease and likely have a shorter lifespan.

Fortunately for Dr. Wahls, she wasn't willing to accept this prognosis. She knew from her academic medical training that the latest discoveries in the research world take at least twenty to thirty years to filter down into conventional clinical practice. So, she started doing her own research, and began making a list of nutrients that had been shown to be beneficial for brain health, and thus might help her condition. She also discovered Functional Medicine and began to think about her condition in completely different terms. What if there was a way not only to slow the progression of her disease but reverse it?

In December of 2007, Dr. Wahls began a dietary and supplement protocol based on her exhaustive research. The results stunned her physician, her family, and Dr. Wahls herself: within a year, she could walk through the hospital without a cane and even completed an eighteen-mile bicycle tour. She went from being in a wheelchair to walking and bicycling without support in *less than twelve months*.

Over the next several years, Dr. Wahls refined and expanded her protocol, and then introduced it to the public in her book *The Wahls Protocol: A Radical New Way to Treat All Chronic Autoimmune Conditions Using Paleo Principles* (Wahls 2014). Since then, thousands of people around the world have successfully treated their autoimmune conditions—not just MS, but other autoimmune problems like inflammatory bowel disease, Hashimoto's, and rheumatoid arthritis—with the Wahls protocol.

This is remarkable given that the conventional approach to treating autoimmune disease is almost exclusively focused on suppressing and managing symptoms. For example, if Farah has rheumatoid arthritis, she might be prescribed steroids to reduce inflammation, and analgesics to relieve pain. These drugs often have side effects, such as weight gain and constipation, so Farah may also end up taking additional drugs to deal with these side effects. Before long, Farah is taking five to six medications—which she'll need to take for the rest of her life—without any true change in her condition.

With a Functional Medicine approach to autoimmune disease, such as the Wahls protocol, Farah has the potential to not only stop the progression of her disease, but in some cases to reverse it completely. What's more, she can do this with diet, supplements, and lifestyle changes, avoiding the adverse effects and long-term risks that come with immunosuppressive drugs and pain relievers. Functional Medicine offers hope and real transformation to patients like Farah, who would otherwise be consigned to a lifetime of medications, doctor's visits, and suffering.

Patient's Perspective

GERD

Let's see how Functional Medicine works differently from the conventional approach. We'll start with Ashley, who suffers from GERD, or reflux. GERD affects a shockingly high number of people—statistics suggest that 20 to 30 percent of Americans suffer GERD symptoms weekly (Zhao and Encinosa 2008). For as long as she has dealt with this problem, Ashley has been told to treat her reflux with proton pump inhibitors, or PPIs. PPIs were only approved by the FDA for short-term use of two weeks or less, but that recommendation has been widely disregarded; some people have been on them for decades. Unfortunately, PPIs can lead to all sorts of problems. PPIs work by completely suppressing stomach acid production. These drugs are remarkably effective at achieving that goal, and can significantly reduce reflux and other symptoms of GERD. The problem is that they don't do anything to address the cause of the acid refluxing into the esophagus in the first place. What's more, they have numerous adverse effects. First, stomach acid plays many important roles in the body—it's not just there to give us heartburn. It protects us against infectious organisms that might be present in things we eat and drink, and it helps with the absorption and assimilation of protein, vitamins, and minerals. Second, proton pumps aren't limited to the stomach; they're present in just about every cell in the body, and they're involved in the process of cellular energy production. This explains why PPIs are associated with numerous adverse effects, from altering the gut microbiota, to impairing nutrient absorption, to increasing the risk of cardiovascular events, to damaging the kidneys, to decreasing cognitive function (Kresser 2016).

As serious as these side effects can be, the worst problem with PPIs is that they may contribute to the very problem that they're meant to solve. Ashley's test results revealed that she had SIBO. Research has shown that SIBO may be an underlying cause of GERD, and PPIs may increase the risk of SIBO (Tziatzios et al. 2017). I treated Ashley with botanicals, probiotics, and other nutrients to address her SIBO, and I also suggested she follow a diet low in certain types of carbohydrates that serve as a food source for the bacteria in the small intestine.

Within three weeks, Ashley completely stopped taking her PPI—after years of using it daily—and she reported an 80 percent reduction in her symptoms. For the first time in recent memory, she was having full days where she didn't experience any GERD symptoms at all, and even when she did experience them, they were much less severe and shorter-lived. If you or someone close to you has suffered from GERD, you know how debilitating and life-altering it can be and how welcome an improvement like this would be. Ashley was truly ecstatic and felt as if her life had been given back to her.

PROBLEMS WITH PPIS

Over the last two decades, studies have shown that PPIs can increase the risk of infection and significantly increase nutrient deficiency (Kresser 2016). One nutrient particularly stamped out by PPIs is B12, which is crucial for cognitive health—and indeed, several studies have found an association between PPIs and cognitive health. There's also a strong association between PPI use and bone fractures in the elderly. PPIs have been shown to increase the risk of cardiovascular events because they reduce the production of nitric oxide, a substance that promotes the dilation of blood vessels and improves blood flow. Elderly people who have been on PPIs for many years often suffer from osteoporosis, cardiovascular disease, and cognitive problems. The general assumption is that these issues are simply a result of getting older—but PPIs (and other medications) are likely to play a significant role in the conditions that we associate with older age.

Migraines and neuropathy

Eric, a patient with severe neurological conditions, came to the clinic after seeing a primary care doctor, several neurologists, and other specialists. He suffered from tics and tremors, neuropathy, migraines, and visual disturbances. The doctors Eric saw had run several tests specific for neurological function but were unable to offer him a diagnosis that went beyond a description of his symptoms. They prescribed several different medications with the aim of providing relief, but unfortunately, none were effective (and most had intolerable side effects).

In our initial appointment, I explained to Eric that his symptoms may be related to problems in his gut, which his previous doctors hadn't tested for. Eric was understandably skeptical, since he didn't have any digestive symptoms. But he was desperate to find an answer, so he agreed to do some additional testing.

The results indicated that Eric had undiagnosed celiac disease (CD). Most people—including doctors—think that celiac disease is exclusively a digestive disorder. Research tells a different story. One in two patients diagnosed with CD does not have gut symptoms, and for every diagnosed case of CD, there are 6.4 cases that remain undiagnosed (Fasano and Catassi 2001)—most of which are atypical or silent forms with no gut symptoms (Catassi et al. 1995). Celiac disease has been linked with a wide variety of diseases outside of the intestine, such as type 1 diabetes, multiple sclerosis, heart failure, depression, arthritis, and dermatitis. This explains why CD can manifest with symptoms outside of the digestive tract, ranging from chronic headaches to dermatitis to joint pain to insomnia (Kresser 2013a).

When Eric removed gluten from his diet, his migraines, tics, tremors, and other symptoms stopped. He recovered about 95 percent of his previous function. How is this possible? How could a condition characterized by intolerance to a single food substance cause migraines, neuropathy, and tremors? Celiac disease damages the intestinal barrier and causes it to become permeable. When this happens, large proteins and toxins produced by gut microbes escape the gut and enter the bloodstream where they provoke a chronic, low-grade inflammatory response. This inflammation then affects organs and tissues throughout the body, including—in Eric's case—the brain and the nervous system.

Fortunately, in Eric's case, the solution was remarkably simple. We found a single underlying cause: gluten. A single dietary element had triggered a cascade of symptoms in different parts of his body. Eric had seen different doctors for different symptoms, and they all offered different drugs to treat those symptoms. Nobody was thinking systematically about a *single cause* that could produce all these symptoms. That's the difference between the dualistic approach of conventional medicine and the more holistic approach of Functional Medicine.

Camila is another example. She came to see me because she and her husband had been unable to conceive for the past three years, despite using in vitro fertilization (IVF) and other assisted reproductive technologies. This is unfortunately a common problem; recent statistics suggest that about one in eight couples have trouble getting pregnant (CDC 2016).

In the conventional paradigm, little attention is given to investigating the underlying causes of infertility. Treatments typically involve drugs to stimulate ovulation, hormone injections, or IVF, in which fertilized eggs are placed in the woman's uterus. Although these interventions may be effective, they do not address the reason why the couple is unable to conceive in the first place.

In Functional Medicine, we start by asking *why* the couple is having trouble getting pregnant. The possibilities include nutrient deficiency, thyroid problems, sex hormone imbalance, inflammation, insulin resistance and blood sugar abnormalities, chronic stress, and environmental toxins—to name a few. Since infertility may be related to either partner, it is often necessary to test both to determine what the underlying issues are.

In Camila's case, we found that both her and her husband

were suffering from chronic mercury toxicity that resulted from an extended overseas stay in China, where they were both working. Studies have found that higher blood mercury levels are correlated with infertility in both men and women (Choy et al. 2002). We started a mercury detox protocol with both Camila and her husband, and three months after their mercury levels had normalized, they successfully conceived. What's more, they did this without any assisted reproductive technology. Nine months later, Camila delivered a healthy baby girl. She was in tears when we spoke on the phone; she felt that she might have missed her chance to have a biological child had she not discovered Functional Medicine and learned that hidden mercury toxicity was preventing her from conceiving. Unfortunately, issues like these are all too common—and most often go undiscovered.

As a practitioner, there's nothing that gives me more joy than helping a couple to conceive and bring a healthy child into the world, especially when either partner has been told that they're "infertile." I've learned over time not to believe this diagnosis, since in many cases the couple is able to conceive once the underlying causes of "infertility" have been addressed.

Where to Start?

Although the "inside, out" paradigm is our most consistent approach, there are times when it's necessary to begin care by immediately addressing the outermost ring. Let's consider Dylan, a patient with a truly confounding set of symptoms, stemming from what is often a confounding disease: Lyme. Perhaps Dylan had come in for his first appointment at our clinic and said, "I was bitten by a tick two days ago. I removed it and now I've got this bull-seye rash, and I'm having neuropathy and night sweats and fever." If that were the case, we obviously would not start with diet and lifestyle. We would immediately begin treating Dylan's infection.

But what if Dylan's case wasn't so easy to address? What if Dylan never remembers getting bitten by a tick, but has tested positive for Lyme and been treated with antibiotics by another practitioner? What if, even after taking all those antibiotics, Dylan continues to have symptoms? In his first consultation with us, Dylan might describe the frustrating journey it's been: "First, they said I had Lyme, then after I didn't get better with treatment, they told me I don't have Lyme, and that it's some other syndrome. I think they called it 'post-treatment Lyme disease syndrome,' whatever that's supposed to mean. One doctor said it was chronic Lyme, but then another doctor said chronic Lyme isn't even real. I don't know what's going on."

Lyme disease is still a mystery. Initially, the CDC stressed that chronic Lyme didn't exist. If a person got a tick bite and had Lyme, he was supposed to take antibiotics for Lyme and that would be the end of the story. There have been some chinks in the armor of that hypothesis recently. Researchers such as Professor Ying Zhang at Johns Hopkins University have shown that *Borrelia*, the bacterium that causes Lyme disease, can persist in forms that are resistant to commonly used antibiotics. This suggests that chronic Lyme may exist after all, and there are many instances where people who have been treated for chronic Lyme have improved.

In a situation like Dylan's—where there's much still to be discovered and new research that questions earlier assumptions—where do we begin in the functional model?

The Functional Medicine Pyramid

Discerning the most effective way to structure and layer a patient's treatment is part of the practice of Functional Medicine. Even as we consider all possible points of intervention in a complex patient's case like Dylan's, we must identify a starting place. The Functional Medicine pyramid below illustrates what I've found to be the optimal progression of treatment for most patients. There are exceptions, such as with a patient with an acute infection that needs to be addressed immediately, but the pyramid can help us walk through the most common, and often most useful, progression.

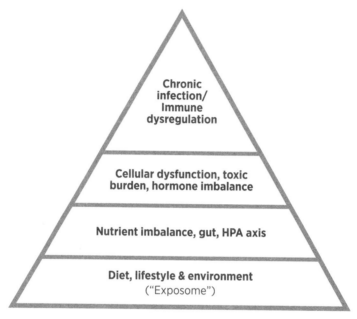

The Functional Medicine Pyramid

We almost always start with the foundational layer—diet, lifestyle, and environment. That's especially true for chronic illnesses. If Dylan were a patient at our clinic, we would likely start with the bottom two levels of the pyramid. If the foundation is shaky, whatever we do to address the Lyme—if that is indeed the issue—is going to be less effective. In Dylan's case, we would start with gut health, nutrients, HPA axis (hypothalamic pituitary adrenal axis, the system of the body that governs our response to and is most affected by stress), diet, and lifestyle. Patients often experience significant improvement by addressing these areas alone. Only after the foundation is established do we go on to address infections and other issues higher in the pyramid.

We use this pyramid approach with most patients' conditions. If a patient comes in with an autoimmune disease or gives us a long list of symptoms with no clear cause, then we make our way up the pyramid. In most cases, we begin at the bottom of the pyramid because we know from clinical experience and from research that those areas are likely to have the biggest impact on the broadest range of conditions.

Why does an inside, out, bottom-up approach work so well on modern, chronic disease? It's because of what drives those diseases—the mismatch between modern diet, lifestyle, and environment and our basic human biology. This mismatch is the primary driver of chronic disease. What our bodies need, ancestrally speaking, is not what our bodies get in the modern world. In the next chapter, we'll look at this in more detail.

CHAPTER NINE

REALIGNMENT: MATCHING OUR ENVIRONMENT WITH OUR GENES

The second element of the ADAPT Framework is an ancestral diet and lifestyle, which is based on the premise that we must bring our environment into closer alignment with our genes to thrive. Humans evolved in a vastly different environment than the one we're living in now. We like to think of ourselves as somehow exempt from the rules that govern evolutionary biology, but, in fact, we're not. We're an organism just like any other organism, and we're subject to the same evolutionary principles.

The environment has changed dramatically in the last 10,000 years. Our first huge shift took us from hunter-gatherers to farmers, and then we took another massive leap into the Industrial Revolution. Even in the last fifty to 100 years, our world has changed in profound ways. Genes typically take hundreds or thousands of years to change; they simply cannot keep up with the pace of environmental change. Approximately 10 percent of our genes have shown signs of adaptation since the dawn of agriculture, while 90 percent are the same as they were during the hunter-gather period, which represents most of human evolution (Williamson et al. 2007). It's unlikely our genes will ever adapt to thrive on donuts and Doritos. Those foods simply don't have the nutrients we need to operate. It's hard to imagine what genetic adaptations we'd have to pull off for our genes to function optimally on sugar with no other nutrients. Our modern diet is plainly not designed for our optimal functioning or good health.

So, what do we do? We can't avoid our modern environment altogether. Instead, we need to better align our diet, lifestyle, and environmental exposures with our genes and biology. This doesn't mean sleeping in the backyard in a loin cloth (although if you want to, you can!). It does mean examining the past for ideas that will help us generate hypotheses for what might be helpful today.

For example, in Chapter Five, I pointed out that humans lived in sync with the natural rhythms of light and dark until roughly 100 years ago when artificial light became commonplace. Other more recent changes, such as a growing number of people working indoors during the day and working night shifts, have also profoundly affected our exposure to light. This led to several unanticipated—and undesirable—impacts on our health. Our genes are hard-wired for the twenty-four-hour light-dark cycle. When we don't get enough exposure to sunlight during the day, or we have too much exposure to artificial light at night, we experience a "mismatch" between our genes and our environment.

It's worth studying mismatch examples like these to identify a clear difference in our modern and ancestral environment. Once we note the change, we can evaluate it to determine if it has a significant impact on human health. We can use this lens on every part of our lives: how we eat, how we sleep, how we move and exercise, and how we live in social environments. For example, if you think about the way humans lived for most of their history—in tribal social arrangements—you might notice how different the modern nuclear family is. Even in the industrialized world, most of our grandparents or great-grandparents were still living in extended family arrangements. How has the shift affected our health?

Keeping our evolutionary context in mind helps us to identify areas of profound difference to research further. Once it's been established that there is indeed a problem stemming from the "mismatch," then we can use the ancestral template to generate ideas for how to move closer to our healthiest lifestyle within our current circumstances. This approach will not only help manage chronic illness, but it will also allow us to thrive in our environment and even prevent and reverse disease.

The modern diseases that countless people suffer from today, like heart disease, diabetes, and many autoimmune diseases, are nearly nonexistent in hunter-gatherer populations. It's tempting to think that's because hunter-gatherers didn't get old enough to develop those diseases, but this isn't true. The average lifespan of people living in Paleolithic hunter-gatherer cultures was shorter than our average lifespan today, but those averages don't take into consideration the much higher rates of infant mortality and premature deaths from trauma, warfare, exposure to the elements, and complete lack of emergency medical care. Anthropologists have found that when hunter-gatherer cultures have access to even the most rudimentary form of emergency medical care, like a clinic half-a-day's hike away, they live lifespans that are roughly equivalent to our own, particularly if they're living in a relatively secure, peaceful environment (Gurven and

Kaplan 2007). The difference between these contemporary hunter-gatherers and us is they reach old age without acquiring the plethora of chronic modern diseases that we suffer from in the industrialized world.

Deconstructing "Paleo"

You've probably heard of the "Paleo" or "caveman" diet, which reduces the concept of evolutionary realignment to a couple of handy catchwords. It's helpful to have a shorthand—a common vocabulary—for talking about this paradigm; but these buzzwords don't tell the whole story. Worse, the concept can seem ridiculous without context. People say, "Why would we go back to a diet or lifestyle that our distant ancestors ate and lived? We are the most advanced civilization so far, so why would I want to go back to living in a cave?" Many people hear "Paleo," and immediately tune out, mistakenly thinking we're asking them to give up modern conveniences and pleasures.

Some critics of Paleo have pointed out that it's a flawed concept because our Paleolithic ancestors did not eat the same diet; there was no single "Paleo diet." This is true—at least to some extent. The traditional Inuit, for example, ate a very different diet than people living in the South Pacific—like the Kitavans, or the traditional Okinawans, or the Tukisenta living in Papua New Guinea.

The traditional Inuit lived in the Arctic where they consumed an inordinately high proportion of calories from fat and ate few carbohydrates. They ate what was available. If we looked solely at their diet and concluded, "This is representative of a Paleo diet," then we would begin consuming 80 percent of our calories from fat, avoiding carbohydrates, and looking to buy seal blubber from our grocery store deli. This seems laughable, but some people have used the ancient Inuit diet as a way of justifying a low carbohydrate approach without considering that the Inuit ate that way not by choice but because that's all they had access to. During the summer, when the ice melted, the Inuit consumed whatever plant foods were available, including berries, tubers, roots, stems, and grasses. They also traded for these foods whenever possible.

Likewise, we can't make inferences about what a typical Paleo diet is from looking at the diet of the Tukisenta, who eat mostly sweet potatoes. Ninety-seven percent of their diet comes from sweet potatoes, or from carbohydrates developed from sweet potato. The other 3 percent describes the small amount of fat and protein the Tukisenta get from the insects on the sweet potatoes (Trowell and Burkett 1981). Yet we would be mistaken to conclude, "Well, I guess we should cut out everything in our diets except sweet potato." It would be foolish to make such a sweeping conclusion based on our review of a single group.

Along the same lines, the idea that no Paleolithic people ate grains or legumes has been recently challenged. Archeological evidence reveals that people consumed grain and legumes well before the dawn of the agricultural revolution (Henry et al. 2010). These foods may not have been staples, but people were harvesting them and eating them. This rigid idea that Paleolithic people didn't eat any grains or legumes is probably not true.

Yet as varied as diets were among Paleolithic cultures, **they had far more commonalities than differences.** One ate blubber and another sweet potatoes, but none of them ate Twinkies or Twizzlers. Not one of them guzzled Caramel Crunch Frappuccino's. Modern processed, refined, and sugar-filled foods, so ubiquitous in the average American's diet, were completely absent in the diet of our ancestors and continue to be absent in the diet of contemporary hunter-gatherers. Every hunter-gatherer culture that we know of ate some combination of unprocessed, unrefined foods: meat, fish, fruits and vegetables, nuts and seeds, starchy tubers and roots, and in rare cases, small amounts of legumes and perhaps whole grains.

Our environment has changed, but our genes have not.

Evolution and Epigenetics

When understood correctly, the Paleo approach seeks to align our genes and biology with our epigenome—our genes' response to our environment. Evolutionary biology explains that all organisms—from the simplest single-celled organisms up to the most complex, multicellular organisms—evolved to survive and thrive in a species-appropriate environment. Certain types of bacteria can only survive in extreme environments, like a hydrothermal vent. They've evolved to survive in those environments, eating food only found in those environments. If those bacteria were removed from their extreme conditions and dropped into a shallow ocean, they wouldn't survive.

In other words, if their environment changes more quickly than they can adapt, they're not going to last. Even if they make it, they're still unlikely to thrive.

Think about cats as an example. Cats are true carnivores. Their digestive tract and physiology evolved in response to eating exclusively animal products. If a cat eats grains and other foods unsuitable for a carnivore, they get sick and fail to thrive. You might have noticed that most higher quality cat foods have labels that say, "meat-only diet." Advertisers promote that because veterinarians and zoologists have acknowledged that cats are carnivores, and it's inappropriate to feed them a grains and kibble-type of diet. (Strangely, many pet owners have begun feeding their animals a more "genetically-aligned" diet, yet they haven't yet embraced a similar approach for themselves.)

Humans aren't carnivores like cats; we're omnivores. This means we can eat both animal products and plant foods. But while it's true that there's a wide variation in what human beings can eat, that doesn't mean we can eat anything we want without consequence. We still require adequate amounts and the right types of macronutrients like protein, fat, and carbohydrate. More importantly, we need a long list of micronutrients like vitamins, minerals, and trace minerals to function properly. The industrialized diet is low in many of these micronutrients, which explains why **nearly one-third** of the U.S. population is deficient in at least one essential vitamin or mineral (Bird et al. 2017).

Our biology is defined not just by our genes but also how those genes express, a concept known as epigenetics. Epigenetics describes changes that may occur to a chromosome, which affect gene activity and expression but not the underlying genes themselves. We've learned a lot about epigenetics over the last twenty years or more. We thought we inherited genes from our parents, passed them down to our kids, and that was that. We know now that epigenetics is probably much more important than the genes themselves, in terms of determining our susceptibility to chronic disease and our health over our entire lifespan.

EPIGENETICS IN ACTION

Mice raised by stressed mothers are more likely to be stressed themselves. Stress causes changes in DNA methylation that affect receptors for cortisol, a major stress hormone. So, the offspring of these mothers have a biological susceptibility to stress that was "pre-programmed" by exposure to a stressful environment early in their life.

Studies in rats have shown that exposure to bisphenol-A (BPA, a chemical in plastics and receipts) causes significant reproductive problems, including declines in fertility, sexual maturity, and pregnancy success. Disturbingly, the effect is more pronounced in the third generation—that is, the first generation of rats not directly exposed to the chemical—than in the exposed rat or its offspring (Ziv-Gal et al. 2016).

These are examples of changes to our genes that aren't related to changes to the underlying genetic code itself. They suggest that the choices we make around food, lifestyle, and behavior don't just affect us, they may also affect our children and grandchildren.

An Ancestral Diet & Lifestyle

Our diet, our social environment, the water we drink, the air we breathe, pharmaceuticals we take, or chemicals we're exposed to—each of these exposures affects how our genes express. That critical interaction is what really determines whether we're sick or healthy; it determines how long we live, and our quality of life across the board. When we discuss an ancestral diet, we're talking about an approach that will profoundly affect how our genes express, leading them to ultimately express in a way that brings us toward health, wellness, and longevity. The epigenetic expressions prompted, however, by our modern environment, diet, and lifestyle lead us toward disease and shortened lifespan.

This concept can be illustrated by looking at methylation, which involves the addition of a methyl group (one carbon atom bonded to three hydrogen atoms) to a DNA molecule. We know that several factors—from the food we eat to the chemicals that we're exposed to—can impact methylation of DNA. We also know that methylation of DNA strongly affects our susceptibility to cancer. Methylation can either turn genes on or it can turn them off. As certain genes get turned on by methylation, that can lead to cancer.

Food

The evolutionary perspective is vital, therefore, as we consider the effect of diet and lifestyle on our epigenetics. For 77,000 generations, the human diet consisted primarily of meat and fish, some wild fruits and vegetables, nuts and seeds, and some starchy plants, which varied regionally. All of those are whole foods. They're nutrient-dense. They're packed with micronutrients, vitamins and minerals, antioxidants, and they're relatively low in calories. Most of these foods contain high amounts of water and fiber, which makes us feel full when we eat them.

In contrast, the diet we eat today is the opposite. **We went from eating nutrient-dense, naturally low-calorie, anti-inflammatory food, to eating nutrient-depleted, calorie-dense, pro-inflammatory food.** It's jaw-dropping to think about how drastically we've parted from dietary alignment.

Sleep

Sleep is another area where we have far distanced ourselves from the habits humans practiced for most of history. We evolved in a natural cycle of light and dark, with no artificial light. When the sun went down, it was dark, and when the sun came up, there was light. People generally got at least seven to eight hours of sleep a night. Today, one-third of Americans get fewer than six hours of sleep, up from just 2 percent in 1960 (Knutson et al. 2010). One reason for this is that people are exposed to artificial light at night when their bodies are naturally programmed to need sleep. They may also spend most of the day inside of an office, and thereby miss exposure to sunlight at the biologically appropriate times. We also make demands on our bodies that are far out of joint with what we evolved to experience. We travel across time zones. We work night shifts or rotating shifts that disrupt our circadian rhythms. Forcing our bodies to sleep and wake in such unnatural patterns unmistakably impacts human physiology, leading to associations with all kinds of different diseases, from obesity, to cancer, to heart disease.

Movement

Our physical habits are also a far cry from what they were for most of human existence. Humans have been naturally active throughout history. Hunter-gather societies walked an average of 10,000 steps a day, and that walking was punctuated by briefer periods of more intense physical activity, like chasing down prey. Nobody sat down for long. Some contemporary hunter-gatherers, like the Aché in Paraguay, the Tsimané in Bolivia, and the Hadza in Africa, still live this way. It's no surprise, then, that the rates of chronic disease in these populations are much lower than they are in the industrialized world. (We'll learn more about the Tsimané in Chapter Eleven.)

Social Life

For most of human history, even up until about fifty to seventy years ago, humans lived in close-knit tribal and social groups, with multiple generations. This is how humans still live in many parts of the developing world. But in the modern industrialized world, we live in isolated nuclear family living arrangements. This relative isolation has arguably led to negative effects on our health and well-being. In fact, lack of social support is a bigger predictor of early death than body mass index, blood pressure, and even smoking up to fifteen cigarettes a day (Holt-Lunstad et al. 2010). Social support is one more aspect of modern society that has drifted from our ancestral context, and may be significantly impacting our health.

Work and Play

Many studies of hunter-gatherer societies determined that they generally "worked" about three to four hours a day—and in most cases, "work" meant hunting. Furthermore, their work required skill and intelligence, was carried out in a social context, and it wasn't compulsive. Hunting, gathering, building shelter, or other work required for living might take up three to four hours a day, although some populations worked longer than that. Still, there was ample time for leisure activities, including games, ceremonies, music, singing, dancing, traveling to other bands to visit friends and relatives, and even time for lying around and relaxing. In many ways, the life of the typical hunter-gatherer looks a lot like the modern life of someone on vacation!

Modern Lifestyle = Modern Disease

Our modern lifestyle retains little of our history. We eat differently, we sleep differently, we move, relate, and work differently. Not surprisingly, these changes have had an enormous impact on our health. The way we live has led to chronic inflammation, which we now know is at the root of most modern diseases—including heart disease, diabetes, obesity, autoimmune disease, Alzheimer's, Parkinson's, and many others.

Inflammation is a natural and normal process; in fact, we need it to heal. For example, if I get a cut on my hand, that area will become inflamed. The white blood cells and all the healing substances in my body travel through the blood to that area to protect the wound from any foreign organisms that might enter it and cause infection. The rush of the healing organisms leads to inflammation and simultaneously works to heal that area. Inflammation itself is not bad or evil; we need it to survive. But when inflammation happens inappropriately or doesn't resolve, we have a problem.

In the case of my cut, the inflammation only lasts a short

while. It does what it's supposed to do, and then it resolves. In the diseases named above, the inflammation becomes chronic. The normally protective immune system starts to cause damage to its own tissues, so the body responds as if normal tissues are infected or abnormal.

This kind of runaway inflammation can happen everywhere in our body. It can happen in the joints, which causes arthritis. It can happen in the arteries and vessels, which can cause cardiovascular diseases, heart disease, stroke, and so on. It can happen in the brain, which can cause Parkinson's, dementia, and Alzheimer's, and contribute to a wide range of neurological conditions, many of which are on the rise, like MS. It can happen in the endocrine organs, like the thyroid, adrenal glands, and ovaries, which can lead to conditions like hypothyroidism, Addison's disease and premature ovarian failure. It can happen in the gut, which might lead to functional problems like IBS, more serious structural conditions like Crohn's disease or ulcerative colitis, and even conditions outside the gut such as Parkinson's, Alzheimer's, depression, ADHD, and autism spectrum disorder.

Chronic inflammation is insidious; it often affects multiple tissues. If someone is eating an inflammatory diet and living an inflammatory lifestyle, that could cause a wide range of symptoms, like headaches, brain fog, difficulty sleeping, digestive issues, and joint pain. The conventional model views these symptoms as unrelated; a patient might see a gastroenterologist for the digestive issues, a rheumatologist for the joint pain, and a neurologist for the headaches and brain fog. In Functional Medicine, we recognize that these diverse symptoms often share a common root cause: inflammation.

There are many genetic predispositions that make some people more susceptible to inflammation, and to certain inflammatory processes. Yet whether they develop a disease depends entirely on epigenetics—the interaction of their genes with environmental factors. That disease won't put down roots and grow unless it gets both water and sunlight—in this case, the genetic predisposition, plus the environmental influence. The combination of the two is what leads that gene to express, and create its negative impact.

Some people assume genetic predisposition is everything. But if a man's mother has diabetes, he's not destined to develop it. Our fate isn't written in stone. Our genes are largely the same as they were during the Paleolithic era. If our health came down entirely to our genetic makeup, then contemporary hunter-gatherer populations would have all the same diseases that abound in the United States today. But these populations are remarkably lean and fit and virtually free of the chronic diseases that plague the industrialized world.

Even in the U.S., obesity has only become epidemic over the last fifty years. In 1960, just 13 percent of Americans were obese, compared to nearly 37 percent today. That's a nearly three-fold increase in just half a century. There's no way our genes alone can explain this. Fifty years is simply not enough time for such meaningful changes to occur.

Our genetic predisposition does seem to determine overall susceptibility to the modern lifestyle. We've all met the person who can eat a terrible diet, burn the candle at both ends, and yet still appear to be relatively unaffected. Some people are simply more resilient and better able to tolerate the effects of the modern lifestyle. Others are not so fortunate.

Genetic predispositions can also manifest in different ways. Let's imagine taking ten hunter-gatherers from different places all around the world, and then switching them to a modern diet and lifestyle. They're not all going to develop the same diseases. One person might develop heart disease, another diabetes, and another rheumatoid arthritis. That's exactly what happens in our culture. Not everybody develops the same disease from the same exposures. It's the unique combination of genetics, epigenetics, and the specific environmental influences a person is exposed to from conception that ultimately determines that person's state of health.

CHAPTER TEN

THE 21ST CENTURY PRACTICE: A COLLABORATIVE MODEL

Our current medical model is clearly broken. The conventional system is buckling under the weight of misaligned incentives, broken payment models, inefficiency and bureaucracy, and a paradigm that is not well-suited to address chronic disease. As we've seen, patients don't get enough time with the doctor, nor receive enough support in between appointments. Clinicians are dissatisfied with their inability to provide high-quality care to their patients and are suffering from disillusionment and burnout.

Functional Medicine enables practitioners to uncover the root causes of patient illness, opening the door to true healing rather than just suppressing symptoms with drugs. An ancestral diet and lifestyle empowers patients to prevent and even reverse disease by changing what they eat and how they live. The third element of the ADAPT Framework is a new medical model that better supports the delivery of both Functional Medicine and diet and lifestyle interventions and addresses the problems that plague our "sickcare" system today.

I call this a collaborative practice model. It consists of several elements. First, it embraces a more streamlined operation, which reduces overhead and bureaucracy and provides a higher level of care for patients and a better work environment for clinicians. Second, it refers to a practice that offers both in-person and virtual (via telephone and video conference) appointments, which gives both patients and practitioners more flexibility and allows practitioners to expand their practice beyond their immediate geographical area. Third, as the name implies, it suggests a model that incorporates both licensed providers, like medical doctors and nurse practitioners, and non-licensed allied providers like nutritionists and health coaches, to provide additional layers of support for patients beyond what they typically receive in today's episodic care model.

Let's take a closer look at what this model looks like in practice.

Independently Operated

Most Functional Medicine practices operate independently. Unlike conventional medical doctors, who must work within the confines of a cumbersome system, Functional Medicine practitioners often work as solo practitioners in private practice, or they belong to a group of physicians practicing together. In either case, Functional Medicine doctors make their own decisions, ranging from how they deliver patient care to billing procedures, business operations, and hiring decisions.

The Micropractice Option

Some Functional Medicine practices choose to function as a micropractice. A micropractice typically consists of just one doctor, who may be assisted by a coach or a nurse practitioner. That's the model that's probably going to work for most clinicians. A micropractice simplifies the primary care office to its most essential components so that it's capable of delivering patient-centered, collaborative care. Functional Medicine focuses on delivering the best quality of care for our patients, and this is often contingent on reduced overhead.

My own clinic is larger, with four clinicians, a nurse practitioner, a health coach, two nutritionists, and thirteen administrative staff, but many of our strategies on reducing overhead lend themselves well to the micropractice model. For instance, we cut costs by not having a large, centralized location with the staff onsite. I sublet an office in a larger office. My personal office is adjacent to a waiting room with aesthetically pleasing furniture and beautiful lighting. It's a restful, peaceful environment. Prior to coming, my patients will have filled out whatever forms they need to fill out online. If they had any questions, they've been answered via phone or email by one of my staff members who's not onsite. They've been given instructions for how to go to the office and what to do when they get there. They wait in this lovely waiting room, have a glass of water or tea, and sit there until I'm ready. After I finish with my previous patient, I walk out into the room, say goodbye to the person I was just meeting with, greet the new patient, and we go back to my office.

If I need to order labs, I can send them to a local blood draw station, which means we don't require an in-house phlebotomist. If I order supplements for my patient, we drop-ship them from a distributor or from our own online store, which means we don't require a large space or additional staff.

This setup is quite different from what clinicians traditionally experience in a large, centralized medical practice. I don't have a huge space to lease and pay for. I don't have a large staff onsite. I can hire people in different locations who work virtually. I don't have to struggle with high expenses or provide a low-quality patient experience. Cutting costs this way can help clinicians earn more without working more, and simultaneously improve the patient experience.

Lean Operation

Within the conventional model, clinicians don't have much autonomy in determining what tests they can order, what treatments they can prescribe, and what they can suggest to patients. Many of the limits come from the rules established by insurance companies. Working with insurers is not only limiting, it's difficult. Sometimes an insurance company will simply refuse to pay for a procedure, treatment, or visit that the physician recommends in the patient's best interest. Interacting with insurers can be frustrating and exhausting. It requires staff whose sole purpose is to deal with the bureaucracy, paperwork, and seemingly arbitrary regulations related to insurance. The experience on the medical end can be maddening.

Many clinicians are choosing to move to a cash-only or

a cash-plus-insurance practice. We operate on the cash-plus-insurance model—if testing can be run through the patient's insurance, we do that. If the patient's insurance doesn't cover it, the bill goes to the patient instead of the clinician; this dramatically reduces the practice's overhead, thereby creating a much "leaner" practice. Within this model, the practitioners are the decision makers in terms of what kinds of testing and treatment they make available to their patients—not a remote insurance company. As you might expect, this has major positive implications for patient care.

Unfortunately, the current lack of insurance coverage for Functional Medicine makes it hard to access for patients without the means to pay for it. I believe that this will change over time. As I argued in Chapter Eight, when the true costs of care (without insurance subsidies) are considered, Functional Medicine is far more affordable than conventional medicine. Later in the book we'll learn how organizations like Cleveland Clinic and Iora Health are demonstrating this, and why it's virtually inevitable that Functional Medicine will become the default model of healthcare in the future.

In the meantime, there are ways that Functional Medicine can be made more accessible. Some practitioners use a sliding scale pay method to help mitigate costs for lower income patients. Others offer discounts for people with financial need. One benefit of a cash-only model is that it enables clinicians to redirect some of the resources that were being used to deal with the insurance bureaucracy, and instead invest in hiring allied providers. Appointment fees with these providers are often lower than with the primary clinicians. Allied providers can also offer group classes and visits, which are more affordable than one-on-one sessions. For these reasons, the cash-only model can have tremendous benefits for patients if they are able to afford the care.

The combination of the leaner operation model and the use of allied providers can also increase the clinician's income potential. If clinicians only make money when they're seeing patients, that puts a hard limit on the amount of revenue that can be earned. If they're also earning a small portion of money when the allied providers are seeing patients or running classes and groups, they can significantly expand their revenue potential without working more hours.

The leaner practice model creates more flexibility and convenience for both patients and practitioners. A cash-only operation can mean less overhead for the clinician, and increased income potential through working with allied providers. The income is valuable, but the improved quality of life clinicians can access in the leaner model is even more rewarding. Clinicians can work fewer hours, spend more time with their families, take care of themselves, make sure they're getting enough exercise, manage their stress, and take vacations without suffering financially. The improved quality of life gives Functional Medicine practitioners the time and energy to continually learn, research, stay current with the most recent evidence and then implement those changes into their practice. Free from the dictates of insurance bureaucracies, they can run their practice with authenticity and purpose.

Longer Appointments

If a Functional Medicine physician—let's call her Dr. Clark—is seeing a patient for the first time, she'll spend anywhere from sixty to ninety minutes with the patient, over five times as long as a first-time patient might expect in the conventional model. With more time, Dr. Clark can talk to her patients about diet and lifestyle, and get their overall sense of what's contributing to their disease or illness. Important information can come up in those conversations. A patient might mention something offhand that doesn't seem particularly relevant to him but raises a red flag for the experienced physician. For example, perhaps Dr. Clark's patient mentions that he's staying up late using the computer. He might not think that's a problem, but Dr. Clark would know that the blue light emitted from those screens can affect melatonin and interfere with sleep, causing a variety of health problems.

Surprising information can come up when you talk with your patients, information you may not get any other way. If Dr. Clark's intake form asked, "How's your digestion?" her patient might have written "fine" on the form. While talking to him, Dr. Clark learns he has serious discomfort after eating, and he has reflux. Perhaps her patient also mentions he has constipation or diarrhea, but he's grown accustomed to it. He says it's no big deal. He's learned to ignore it. These are things the doctor needs to know. Sometimes patients hesitate to write down their problems on those intake forms. The only way doctors will learn about lifestyle practices like alcohol intake may be to talk with them, face-to-face.

Key details about family history also may arise during longer appointments. A patient might casually mention that her mother had rheumatoid arthritis, or her grandmother had her thyroid gland removed. Dr. Clark will recognize that both conditions are related to autoimmunity, something a patient wouldn't necessarily suspect. Because Dr. Clark knows her patient's family history, she decides to initiate testing of her patient's thyroid antibodies to see if she had an autoimmune thyroid disease too.

These "surprises" can often provide important clues to diagnosing a patient's root cause issues, but would typically go unexpressed during a fifteen-minute conventional model consult.

Along with building a framework for understanding the in-depth context of a patient's health, Dr. Clark also builds a relationship with her patients the longer she talks to them. Practitioners love making meaningful connections with their patients. Most of them entered medicine with the hope of having a discernable positive influence on their patients. They want to help people and form a connection with them. Longer initial meetings make deeper relationships possible.

Longer follow-up appointments can help build trust. Patients who are initially reluctant to divulge certain information might feel more comfortable revealing the details as their relationship with the doctor develops. That's why follow-up appointments at Functional Medicine clinics are also longer than follow-up appointments in the conventional model. It may not be until be the third or fourth appointment that the patient finally feels comfortable enough to start revealing some of the critical details needed for a thorough diagnosis.

Limited Patient Count

Those long appointments don't happen by accident. In Functional Medicine, practitioners tend to carry a much smaller patient load than the average primary care doctor. We noted earlier that the average PCP has 2,500 patients. That's way too many to provide a high level of service, especially when many of those patients have chronic, complex illnesses.

Frequently, PCPs enter appointments with patients they haven't seen for months. Imagine such an appointment with a patient called Lucia. Lucia has diabetes and high cholesterol, and is taking two drugs: a statin to lower cholesterol, and metformin to deal with her blood sugar issues. In this new visit, Lucia also complains of joint pain and swelling in her hands and feet. Something else is going on, but what? In a brief appointment, it's going to be enormously challenging to find out. It may be all the doctor can do to properly follow what's happening with the diabetes symptoms, blood sugar management, and cholesterol. Is he likely to also ask about Lucia's dietary and lifestyle choices? He probably doesn't have time.

The PCP is expected to not only accomplish that comprehensive evaluation, but also conduct a thorough intake on the new symptoms to determine contributing factors. After that, he's charged with helping Lucia deal with those symptoms. Finally, the doctor must make a sound diagnosis and establish a good treatment plan. In twelve minutes. That's nearly impossible, especially if the first five minutes of an appointment are spent with greetings and preliminary check-up questions. Doctors typically have a paltry five or six minutes to address new symptoms, prescribe a meaningful diagnostic test to determine the cause, and establish a treatment plan for those symptoms. No wonder these appointments so often result in an apparently efficient treatment: a prescription for a new drug.

Clearly, the current model isn't providing adequate or thorough patient care. Most of the recent studies advocating for a new model of medicine suggest that the maximum number of patients a primary care practitioner can handle, while still delivering a relatively high quality of care, is closer to 1,500 patients, or even 1,000.

Functional Medicine practitioners handle a much smaller caseload, anywhere from 500 to 750 patients, depending on how much additional support they receive from allied providers such as nurse practitioners, physician assistants, nutritionists, and health coaches within the practice. These providers offer an additional layer of support and point of contact for the patient to receive sufficient care. Doctors supported by allied providers can carry more patients than solo practitioners.

Even with a relatively large clinic like mine, we're able to provide a high level of service to our patients because of the support of allied providers. You can decide what level of patients is appropriate for you. You might want to expand so you can see as many patients as possible at your clinic. Or you might prefer a smaller practice, with simpler management and less complexity. In general, Functional Medicine practitioners meet with fewer patients, for longer times, to optimize patient care.

Connection With Patients and True Healing

We've discussed how a lower patient load means clinicians have time to build the relationships that can have a profound effect on care. In some cases, this can lead to breakthroughs that might not otherwise have happened.

I remember working with a patient, Charlotte, who was dealing with a complex, chronic, multi-system illness that was poorly defined. It didn't fit any of the typical diagnostic categories. She experienced severe digestive distress, intense fatigue, insomnia, terrible sleep quality that hadn't responded to any intervention, skin breakouts and rashes, depression, and acute anxiety. She had lost interest in many of her hobbies and pleasures, and when I first started working with Charlotte, her emotional tone was consistently tense. She was focused on the diet, supplements, and extensive treatments that she hoped would lead to her improvement—but maintaining those practices made her feel wound up all the time. For the first few months of working together, we did some testing and determined some underlying issues to address, but the results fell short. Certainly, her outlook was not improving. Her diet was severely restricted, and as a result, she wasn't spending time with her friends. Her world was growing smaller. She felt like she had done so much to try to address her health yet didn't see much of a return.

I intuitively understood Charlotte needed more joy and pleasure in her life. She needed a deeper connection with herself and a more meaningful way of managing stress. The answer for her was probably not going to come from supplements, treatments, or lab tests. We needed to shift gears.

I asked Charlotte to let go of some of the supplements she was taking, many of which had been prescribed by previous practitioners. She had long questioned whether they were helping her anyway, and simply managing the dosing schedule was practically a full-time job. I asked her to let go of some of her dietary rigidity, which she also wasn't sure was helping much. Then, I asked her to make a list of all the things that brought her joy and pleasure.

Her new treatment was to commit to doing at least one of those activities a day.

Essentially, we designed a program for joy and pleasure. Charlotte immediately felt that this approach was right. She was at a point where she had tried so many methods of treatment, both with previous practitioners and myself, that she didn't have much energy to continue in her current direction. But a joy list? That was a plan she could get behind.

Six months later, she seemed like a different person. She looked relaxed. She smiled and laughed more. She appeared less tense, more at ease. Although the "joy plan" didn't resolve all her physical issues, Charlotte appreciated being able to relate to her health in an entirely different way. She felt hope and happiness that she hadn't felt for years. She restarted some of her hobbies and began traveling again. In fact, she even made a career change. Because she felt like the focus on lifestyle and behavior had been so crucial to her improvement and recovery, she decided to become a health coach, hoping to help others through the same methods that helped her.

My intuitive sense of Charlotte's true problem only developed because of the amount of time that we had spent in appointments together. The answer arrived because of the relationship we had developed.

Telemedicine

Seeing patients in person is invaluable, but it's not the only option. Telemedicine can be part of the mix. Admittedly, video may not be the ideal way to maintain a doctor/patient connection. Video meetings, however, are a close second to meeting in person. You can see the patient, they can see you, and you can have a rich conversation. Insurers are beginning to recognize the value of telemedicine; video conferencing is now reimbursed in many states, and others are moving in that direction.

Options like telemedicine offer convenience not only for practitioners but also for patients with busy lives. If a patient in San Francisco wants a thirty-minute appointment in my office in Berkeley, they may prefer to meet by video conference rather than deal with an hour's worth of traffic and the Bay Bridge!

Practitioners love the flexibility telemedicine affords. They can work occasionally from home, or even while traveling. Clinicians can also see patients they wouldn't have even known about in a traditional setting. Telemedicine expands the geographical boundaries beyond the local area. At our clinic, for example, approximately 70 percent of our patients live outside our immediate area. These patients will either drive or fly in for the first appointment and do it in person.

We require that first face-to-face meeting. It's the best way to establish a relationship. After that, patients can do their follow-up appointments via video conference; once a year, we ask them to come back for another in-person appointment. Telemedicine allows patients who can't access the healthcare services they need in their home town to get the help they need, and you have access to a vastly larger pool of potential patients. That contributes to income stability for your clinic, and reduces time spent advertising—it's easy to promote a telemedicine practice using an online platform, such as a blog, podcast, website, or a social media outreach effort. In fact, this is the only "advertising" I have ever done for my practice, which has been closed to new patients for the better part of the last several years due to high demand and low turnover.

MDHQ

One area of dissatisfaction and pushback among doctors is with electronic health records (EHRs). Initially, there was a lot of enthusiasm for EHRs, but the way they've been implemented in conventional medical settings has been horrific. There's a steep learning curve, and some software has *increased* error rates. A lot of doctors don't like having to look at a screen the whole time they're with a patient.

But those problems are solvable. We use an electronic health record called MDHQ, which is specifically designed for Functional Medicine and for this type of practice. It's streamlined. It doesn't contain a whole bunch of features and things that you don't need in a Functional Medicine practice. It's also got a patient portal, where the patient can access their record. It has a lot of features that make it easier to get things done without having to stare at the computer the whole time you're with a patient.

Collaborative Care Model

Physician appointments are only one part of providing care. The ADAPT Framework also employs a team of allied providers in a collaborative care model. Here's how it works: During a patient's initial appointment with the clinician, he or she would likely receive several recommendations about diet and lifestyle. A small percentage of people easily take those recommendations and run with them independently. Most don't know how. To help patients implement those recommendations, the clinician will suggest a follow-up appointment with a coach, a nurse practitioner, or a physician assistant. These allied providers can spend more time with patients reviewing the nuts and bolts of behavior change and making a plan for the patient to reach his or her goals. Allied providers also follow up with patients regularly for brief check-ins to help them adhere to their lifestyle changes.

In our practice, a patient first meets with a nurse practitioner via phone or video. The nurse practitioner (NP) collects important information from patients, such as why they want to be seen, what their main complaints are, what they've tried so far, what's worked and hasn't worked, what other practitioners they've seen, any labs or other testing they've had, and so on. The NP also collects some basic health history, reviews body systems and symptoms, solicits information about diet and physical activity, and asks about exposure to toxins, infections, and other environmental influences.

The information collected during the initial consult with the NP directly informs the first in-person appointment with the patient, which we call the "case review." The clinician reviews the patient's past and present lab testing, detailed intake forms, and health history before entering the room, and prepares a report that outlines the underlying patterns the clinician thinks are contributing to the patient's complaints, recommendations for further testing, and a treatment plan. This approach enables us to see the whole picture and make more rapid progress than in the conventional model.

At the end of the initial case review appointment, the clinician makes a series of recommendations for the patient. The proverbial ball is then handed back to the allied providers. If the patient needs additional support with implementation right away, the health coach can walk them through it and answer any questions they might have. The coach may also offer additional resources for changing diet, exercise, and stress management habits.

Approximately two weeks after the patient starts the treatment protocol, he or she might have a brief fifteen- to thirty-minute check-in with either the nurse practitioner or the health coach. The allied provider asks how the protocol is going and about any challenges that they're having. He or she will then make recommendations for adjusting the approach, and provide much-needed moral support. These check-ins are key to the success of the ADAPT Framework. In a conventional model, or even many Functional Medicine practices, the patient might see the doctor two to four times a year, with no contact in between. The paradigm assumes doctors can simply give you information and you'll go do it. As we know, that rarely works.

The ADAPT Framework assumes the patient needs support, and therefore we set up regular check-ins between the patient and the allied provider. We also have emergency appointments available, so if a situation comes up that the coach isn't licensed to handle—perhaps the patient needs an adjustment of her medication, for example—she can have a timely appointment with the nurse practitioner or other licensed allied provider.

Allied providers can also share their expertise with more than one patient at a time. Some practices hold group visits or classes run by allied providers. For example, a nurse practitioner might teach an eight-week class on pain management for patients dealing with chronic pain. The nurse practitioner and health coach work together to create the curriculum, consisting of diet and lifestyle recommendations, and possibly supplement recommendations. Local patients dealing with pain-related conditions get together weekly, building a community as they discuss different ways to address their pain. Patients feel much less isolated and alone when they realize others share their experience.

Allied providers teaching these classes find them very satisfying. Group offerings give them another way to share their expertise and support their patients. Additionally, these classes provide a meaningful experience for the allied providers and practitioners. Many allied providers say their work is energized by the variety of patient perspectives that come up in these groups.

Health coaches often find working in a Functional Medicine practice more satisfying than maintaining a solo practice. Some coaches enjoy working independently, of course, but many more feel isolated. It can be difficult to build a practice, and many health coaches don't enjoy the business and paperwork component. They may not be particularly entrepreneurial, and they may miss the collegiality of a team.

Working with other allied providers on a Functional Medicine team offers new opportunities for these coaches, including job security and interaction with colleagues. Many are also happy to be free of the tedious work of recruiting new clients. The main problem independent coaches face is what to do when they've reached a plateau with a client. They've worked on diet and lifestyle, but maybe the patient has a chronic illness that requires advanced medical treatments. Where do they turn?

When health coaches work with other licensed clinicians, they can offer more resources to their patients. It's a symbiotic relationship: although clinicians can do lab testing, protocols, and prescriptions, they often don't have the time or training to help the patient implement diet and lifestyle changes. Coaches are fantastic at behavioral support but can't do the necessary testing. Working together, they both get better results.

Finally, working in a Functional Medicine clinic can help affirm a health coach's professional value. Due to the less rigorous health coach certification process, health coaches sometimes feel like they're not recognized as vetted professionals. Working in a clinical situation with doctors and other care providers adds a sense of legitimacy to what health coaches do, which helps coaches receive warranted validation. In our clinic, we have found that adding health coaches to our allied providers' team is a win-win for everyone.

THE ROLES OF THE ALLIED PROVIDERS

Allied providers are crucial members of the Functional Medicine team. These practitioners work together with doctors and other clinicians to provide another layer of support and care for patients. Although Functional Medicine clinics work with a variety of allied providers, some of the most common providers and their roles are:

Nurse Practitioners (NP): Highly trained nurse practitioners, who hold national accredited licenses, can prescribe medication, examine patients, diagnose illness, and provide treatment like a doctor. In many states, they can practice autonomously.

Physician Assistants (PA): Like nurse practitioners, physician assistants can examine, diagnose, and treat patients, as well as prescribe medications, though they must be under the direct supervision of a doctor.

Registered Dietitians (RD): RDs complete extensive course work at the bachelor's level, spend 900–1,200 hours within a dietetic internship through an accredited institution, and have passed a dietetic registration exam.

Certified Nutritional Specialists (CNS): These are practitioners who have completed an advanced degree at the master's or doctorate level from an accredited university in nutrition, plus have completed 1,000 hours of a supervised internship, and passed a rigorous exam administered by the board for certification of nutrition specialists.

Physical Therapists: Physical therapists, highly educated, licensed healthcare professionals who can help patients reduce pain and improve or restore mobility, can be an asset to a Functional Medicine clinic.

Health Coaches: Health coaches work with patients primarily on behavior change, one of the most crucial parts of the Functional Medicine model in preventing and reversing chronic disease. The classification of "coach" is becoming increasingly standardized. National and international certification bodies have defined criteria for what a qualified coach should know and what the certification process should look like.

Collaborative Care for Patients

Let's look at one of our patients, Ryan, who benefited from the collaborative approach. He came to see me for a variety of issues. He was forty pounds' overweight—obese according to the BMI scale. He'd been diagnosed with prediabetes, was getting closer to having diabetic blood sugar levels, had sleep apnea, asthma, and other breathing difficulties, atopic dermatitis with itchy and painful rashes, ulcerative colitis with frequent flare-ups, and insomnia. He was on eight regular medications when I saw him, with inhaler and pain medications added in as necessary.

In Ryan's initial work-up, we determined that his diet was

poor. He was busy and found it hard to eat right. He wasn't exercising or moving regularly, and wasn't doing anything to manage stress. We put him on a nutrient-dense, whole foods diet with modifications for weight loss and auto-immunity, and he managed to lose thirty pounds in the first three months that we worked together. We did gut testing and addressed the issues we found. Then we got him doing some simple stress management techniques and taking some supplements to help with sleep and the effects of stress.

You'll notice I said "we" when describing Ryan's treatment. It wasn't just me, the clinician, delivering care. Ryan worked intensively with our health coach and our nurse practitioner to make these changes. He really got a chance to talk about the issues in his life and get clear on how change would be most effective. We then broke these things down into manageable chunks that he could work with.

The collective support made a huge difference for Ryan, and when he started to make those diet, lifestyle, and behavior changes, his symptoms improved simultaneously. He lost weight and his blood sugar went back to normal levels. His sleep apnea disappeared and he no longer had to use his CPAP machine. His dermatitis scaled back considerably, and he started being able to sleep well even without medication. In that three-month period, he got off seven of the eight medications that he took regularly and hadn't used any of the ones that he took on an as-needed basis.

Collaborative Care for Physicians

Providers like Sherry, the physician we heard from in Chapter Six, can escape burnout by switching to the practice model we've described above. Instead of feeling like a cog in a patient mill, and just handing out prescriptions all day long, Sherry now has the time to talk to her patients about ways to prevent and reverse disease. She can utilize allied providers like health coaches and nutritionists to support her patients in making those changes stick. Her new working environment helps her optimize her own quality of life as well. She's now able to pursue her own interests and incorporate those into her practice. She feels like she's having an impact on patients that she never could have in her previous practice. I've heard the same story from many practitioners who have made the switch.

CHAPTER ELEVEN

REGARDING EVIDENCE

Now that we've examined all three elements of the ADAPT Framework—Functional Medicine, an ancestral diet and lifestyle, and a collaborative practice model—I'd like to address the question of evidence. We often hear the claim that conventional medicine is "evidence-based," whereas approaches like Functional Medicine and an ancestral diet and lifestyle are not. But is this true? Let's take a closer look.

Is Conventional Medicine Evidence-Based?

"It is simply no longer possible to believe much of the clinical research that is published," says Marcia Angell, a former editor of the *New England Journal of Medicine* (Full Measure Staff 2017). She should know! John Ioannidis, an influential researcher from Stanford, published the 2005 paper, "Why Most Published Research Is False," to illuminate this problem (Ioannidis 2005). Ioannidis explains that in many research papers, "Claimed findings may be accurate measures of the prevailing bias." Clearly, Dr. Ioannidis struck a nerve; this paper is now the most widely cited paper ever published in the journal *PLoS Medicine*.

In other words, most published research findings support the status quo; they're not necessarily based on solid evidence. Often, the research that builds on an initial study ends up perpetuating questionable findings. It's like building a house of cards: a paper gets published that references another paper; then, a third paper gets published that references that second paper, which referenced that first paper, and so on. The assumption is that the evidence in that first paper was correct—but what if it's not? The edifice of peer-reviewed research is not as perfect as we tend to believe.

Conflicts of interest abound: two-thirds of medical research is funded by pharmaceutical companies (Smith et al. 2014). Such financial ties don't *guarantee* bias, but they do make it more likely. As Upton Sinclair once said, "It's difficult to make a man understand something when his salary depends upon him not understanding it." Sinclair wasn't just imagining this. Studies have repeatedly found that industry-sponsored trials are more likely to report favorable results for drugs because of biased reporting, biased interpretation, or both (Lexchin 2003). The time-honored saying, "Don't bite the hand that feeds you," also applies.

Another problem is that conflicts of interest in academic research are rarely disclosed. A 2009 report issued by the Department of Health and Human Services showed that very few universities required reports to be made to the government about their researchers' financial con-flicts of interest (Levinson 2009). Even when they are reported, the universities rarely require those researchers to eliminate or reduce those conflicts. In fact, 90 percent of universities relied solely on the researchers themselves to decide whether to report their potential conflicts of interest. Half of universities don't ask their faculty to dis-close the amount of money or stock they earn from drug or device makers. True objectivity in scientific research is not as common as we think.

Conflicts of interest aren't just a problem in academia, they're also a problem on advisory panels that influ-ence health policy. In 2008, it was found that eight out of nine of the experts who were responsible for writing the National Cholesterol Education Program Guidelines had ties to statin drug manufacturers (Kresser 2015). Dr. Stephan Guyenet reported in 2008 (Guyenet 2008) that one of the study's authors had, "received honoraria from Merck, Pfizer, Sankyo, Bayer, Merck/Schering-Plough, Kos, Abbott, Bristol-Myers Squibb, and AstraZeneca."

Fraud is also an underappreciated problem in medical research, both intentional and unintentional. Consider a recent paper called "Out of Sight, Out of Mind, and Out of the Peer-Reviewed Literature," published in *JAMA Internal Medicine* (Seife 2015). The study notes that the FDA's findings of fraud in medical research rarely end up being reported. The studies are still published. In this investigation, a researcher falsified a lab test to hide a patient's impaired kidney and liver function in a trial comparing two chemotherapy regimens. The first dose of the regimen proved to be fatal to that patient, and the researcher was ultimately sentenced to seventy-one months in prison. That episode was described by both the FDA and in court documents, but not one of the studies on the chemotherapy trial reported in the peer-reviewed literature made any mention of the falsification of data, the fraud, or the homicide.

INTERVENTIONS WITHOUT EVIDENCE

Many common interventions within conventional medicine are not supported by solid evidence.

Abilify, for example, is one of the best-selling drugs in the United States. It was originally developed as an anti-psychotic, and is approved for schizophrenia, bipolar disorder, depression, and autism spectrum disorders.

The two previous sentences, when taken together, should raise some questions. How could Abilify be one of the best-selling drugs in the country if it's only being used as an anti-psychotic? How many people in this country need an anti-psychotic drug?

Quite a few, it seems. This anti-psychotic drug is now being used for anxiety, ADHD, depression, insomnia, OCD, and to treat all kinds of substance abuse. In fact, 77 percent of the prescriptions given for Abilify are for off-label conditions, meaning there's no evidence supporting the drug's efficacy in treating those conditions. There is also no peer-reviewed scientific evidence to support these uses of Abilify.

The numerous patients taking this drug might experience a wide range of concerning side effects, including weight gain, blurred vision, nausea, vomiting, changes in appetite, constipation, drooling, headache, dizziness, drowsiness, anxiety, sleep problems, and cold symptoms like stuffy nose, sneezing, and sore throat. Yet despite these numerous side effects, and the drug's insubstantial evidence—it continues to be prescribed.

We might hope that the recommendations coming out of conventional medicine offices are all grounded in objective, evidence-based research, but that simply isn't the world we live in.

Functional Medicine's Evidence-Based Approach

In Functional Medicine, we emphasize the importance of evidence-based interventions. If a Functional Medicine clinician tells patients to reduce their exposure to artificial light to help manage their stress, reduce their risk of disease, or even address issues like diabetes and obesity, that's because there's research that supports that connection. We're wary of trends that have no substantial research to back them up.

On the other hand, we also tend to consider new information and methods that are verifiable from evidence earlier than in conventional medicine. Intestinal permeability, or "leaky gut," is a case in point. Twenty-five years ago, the best way to get yourself laughed out of a room full of doctors would have been to start talking about leaky gut—it was considered the realm of alternative quacks. When searching the scientific literature today, the term "intestinal permeability" brings up thousands of articles. Intestinal permeability has been linked to autoimmune disease, diabetes, and depression; certainly, it's a legitimate medical issue that warrants treatment. What seems controversial today may not be so in ten years as new research emerges.

Stomach ulcers are another example. For decades, physicians believed they were caused by stress and perhaps overconsumption of certain foods. Treatment was based on avoiding spicy foods and vague recommendations to manage stress. Then, in the early 1980s, two Australian physicians, Dr. Barry Marshall and Dr. Robin Warren, introduced the idea that ulcers were not caused by stress, but by an infection with a spiral bacterium called *Helicobacter pylori*. Initially, Drs. Marshall and Warren were ridiculed for their unorthodox theory. In fact, it wasn't until Dr. Marshall purposely infected himself with *H. pylori*, developed an ulcer, and then successfully treated it with antibiotics that the scientific community took notice. Even then, more than a decade passed before this new theory became widely accepted, and it wasn't until Drs. Marshall and Warren won the Nobel Prize for Medicine in 2005 that the importance of their discovery was fully acknowledged.

In a hundred years, medical practitioners will probably shake their heads over the methods used today. After all, nobody today would treat a headache by drilling a hole in a patient's head, but that was the practice in the Dark Ages. In fact, it's not an exaggeration to say that the history of science has been the history of *most people being wrong about most things most of the time*. The willingness to challenge even our most deeply held assumptions, and the humility to admit when we've been wrong, are essential to good science. Unfortunately, in the conventional medical paradigm, this willingness and humility have often been replaced by groupthink, arrogance, and a stubborn attachment to the status quo.

In Functional Medicine, we recognize the importance of diagnoses and treatments that are supported by peer-reviewed evidence published in reputable scientific journals. At the same time, we also recognize the real limitations and biases of this research, and we remember that today's heresy may end up being tomorrow's orthodoxy. Therefore, we ground our treatment recommendations both in research and open-mindedness.

Even when we recognize the limits of current research into medicine of any kind, we still ask, what does the research say about Functional Medicine? It's not always easy to tell. Often, Functional Medicine's results are invisible in the scientific literature. Research is conducted in the conventional paradigm of symptom-driven intervention. If you were to search the scientific literature for IBS, for example, you would see several studies supporting the use of Imodium to stop diarrhea; that's symptom-driven research. It would be easy to conclude that Imodium is the best way to treat IBS, even when it isn't.

Functional Medicine is not a symptom-driven model, and

doesn't align readily with symptom-driven research. It's not hard to show that Imodium stops diarrhea. It's much more complex to design a study that demonstrates the efficacy of changing a person's diet, and testing and treating them for SIBO, parasites, or fungal overgrowth. It's harder to design a study that uses multiple interventions customized for each patient. The gold standard of conventional research—the randomized clinical trial—isolates just one variable, then tests the effect of that variable; all other elements of the study are kept the same. The randomized clinical trial is practically the antithesis of the philosophy of Functional Medicine, which seeks to tailor layered treatment plans to individual patients.

The Literature on Functional Medicine

The research supporting the Functional Medicine approach is out there, if you know where to look. Research connects IBS to parasites, to SIBO, to gut-brain axis dysfunction, and to other underlying causes, but those studies are spread across a wide range of publications. You won't find a convenient collection of varied studies on a Functional Medicine approach to IBS in one place.

If a doctor is trying to decide how to treat a patient's IBS, she'll most likely choose the approach that's most accessible. As the PubMed results pile up, she might glance down at her desk and see the brochure on IBS a pharmaceutical sales rep left for her to read. The rep had described a new drug that's been tested and shown to help with IBS, and the brochure lists the latest studies showing the drug's efficacy and benefits. After a long day, it's a relief for this physician to exit out of PubMed and head home, assured that she has found an accepted treatment protocol, which won't require her to scour dozens of individual studies.

Even a better-than-average product like UpToDate (see sidebar) isn't saying, "Here's how you look at this disease from a Functional Medicine approach. Here are the other underlying pathologies that can cause it, and here's how to test for those and treat those."

Attending conferences and continuing education classes can help doctors stay current, but those conferences are often sponsored by a drug company. Much of the information in continuing education is still driven by a corporation with an agenda. Keep your eyes open and you'll find substantial research supporting Functional Medicine.

For example, numerous studies substantiate correlations between IBS and SIBO, along with other gut infections (Bowe and Logan 2011; Daniels et al. 2017; Ghosal et al. 2017). Functional Medicine treatments for psoriasis are well supported by research, too; there's evidence linking skin conditions to changes in gut health and gut flora. Depression has been convincingly linked to systemic inflammation, which in turn is often caused by altered gut microbiota. There is also a vast body of evidence supporting the ancestral diet and lifestyle.

The scientific literature is the most natural place to start when considering new treatments, but it should be tempered with other perspectives as well. Peer-reviewed research is venerated, but in addition to the problems previously addressed, there's an important issue few consider: In many cases, initial research results are never replicated. The scientific method is based on replicability—when there's an initial finding, its value depends on it being reproduced by other researchers in other labs. Typically, a finding isn't considered truly valid until this happens.

Unfortunately, much of the research we've formerly relied upon was never replicated. For example, the Open Science Collaboration tried to replicate 100 published psychology studies under conditions identical to the original research, and 65 percent of the studies failed to replicate the results (Open Science Collaborators 2015). The problem is not just in psychology. In 2011, a group of researchers from Bayer looked at sixty-seven blockbuster drug discovery trials published in prestigious journals; they found that 75 percent of them could not be reproduced (Hartung 2013). Another study of cancer research found that only 11 percent of pre-clinical cancer research could be reproduced (Begley and Ellis 2012).

Does this mean we should throw out all published research altogether? No. Research must be our first step in determining treatment, but we should have a healthy degree of skepticism when consulting scientific publications. This skepticism should lead us to think critically about a study. Perhaps we examine the funding behind a study that seems to endorse a new pharmaceutical with particular zeal. A potential conflict of interest doesn't necessarily mean that the research is invalid, but it's worth investigating.

Functional Medicine physicians often have more time to do that digging. They see fewer patients and therefore have more space in their schedules, and more time to stay current with research. That's important because there's often a big gap between research getting published and when that research trickles down to the practicing PCP. The latest research shows that saturated fat isn't the boogeyman that we thought it might be, but the average PCP is probably not aware of that. If a doctor finds the most current published peer review research in PubMed and asks his colleague if she's familiar with the research, the colleague will likely say no. The latest research often takes time to reach practicing clinicians—and their patients.

UPTODATE

Some databases are better than others, but even the best databases serving most conventional doctors maintain a symptom-driven lens.

UpToDate is a more balanced, subscription-based information product for clinicians. If you look up IBS here, you see an entry describing the treatment of IBS in adults, along with an introduction to the condition, definitions, and indications for referral.

UpToDate is unusual in that it does sometimes talk about dietary therapy, though it moves quickly on to pharmacological therapy, laxatives, how to treat diarrhea, how to treat constipation, and how to treat many other symptoms.

Evidence for an Ancestral Diet & Lifestyle

There are numerous studies in the scientific literature supporting all aspects of the ancestral diet and lifestyle, from the benefits of nutrient-dense, whole foods, to the effects of artificial light on circadian rhythms and sleep, to the need for increased non-exercise physical activity, to the connection between stress and disease, to the importance of play, leisure, and social connection. My first book,

The Paleo Cure, contains over 350 citations documenting these relationships.

For example, the *New York Times* recently published an article about the Tsimané (Brody 2017). They're a subsistence farming and hunter-gather population in Bolivia, who still follow their traditional diet and lifestyle. Researchers went to Bolivia to study heart disease in the Tsimané. They found that the Tsimané's rate of heart disease is about one-fifth of the rate observed in the United States. Nine in ten tribal members had clean arteries and faced no risk of heart disease. An eighty-year-old in the Tsimané group showed the same vascular age as an American in his mid-fifties (Kaplan et al. 2017).

This is important research; it tells us there's clearly something about our diet and lifestyle that's not working. At the same time, it reveals that something about an ancestral diet and lifestyle can help prevent chronic disease (Kresser 2017).

Considering evolutionary alignment is a valid way of generating hypotheses and potentially resolving apparent conflicts in modern research. Consider the Maasai, a tribe in Kenya and Northern Tanzania that gets two-thirds of its calories from fat. They consume 600-2,000 mg of cholesterol a day. In contrast, the American Heart Association (AHA) recommends consuming under 300 mg of cholesterol a day. (As of 2017, the AHA no longer suggests restricting cholesterol intake, due to overwhelming evidence indicating that there is no benefit to doing so.) The Maasai, however, have low blood pressure, low cholesterol, few gallstones, and little atherosclerosis (Bhatia 2012).

If populations like the Maasai achieve low rates of heart disease while eating a high amount of saturated fat, we should question some of our earlier assumptions. A study like this doesn't disprove that saturated fat increases the risk of heart disease on its own but invites us to ask questions. "Is there a different cause for heart disease in modern populations that we haven't considered?" People in the United States with higher rates of heart disease appear to be eating more saturated fat, but that doesn't establish a causal relationship. Maybe there's something else happening. Maybe people who eat more saturated fat are more sedentary, or smoke more, or something else we haven't yet considered. Looking through an evolutionary lens raises these questions.

Observational evidence like this should also spur us to critically examine other research on the topic. When we do that in the case of saturated fat and heart disease, the connection is a lot murkier than the AHA would have you believe. Although saturated fat does raise blood cholesterol levels in some studies, it has no effect in many others (Mensink et al. 2003). More importantly, large reviews have found no direct relationship between saturated fat intake and heart disease (Siri-Tarino et al. 2010), and people who eat more saturated fat have *lower* rates of stroke (Yamagishi et al. 2010). Should we be concerned when saturated fat increases cholesterol if that does not translate into a greater risk of heart disease (and may even reduce the risk of stroke)?

If we look at that data through an evolutionary lens, we're often given needed perspective to generate new ideas for research. We can compare the claim that dietary fat causes heart disease to the experience of traditional populations like the previously mentioned Maasai. When we do, we find inconsistencies. The traditional population consumes a high intake of dietary fat but experiences no heart disease.

Evidence Supporting a Collaborative Practice Model

In the last chapter, we discussed the importance of a collaborative care model, which includes allied providers like nutritionists and health coaches.

Peopie want to feel good, avoid chronic disease, and live

a long life. They want to see their children and grandchildren grow up and have the energy to play with them. They want to perform better at work, enjoy their relationships, and be well enough to get the most out of life. But there's a big difference between wanting the *benefits* of being healthy, and consistently engaging in the *behaviors* that lead to health.

That's where allied providers like health coaches come in. Coaches are trained in several disciplines that support people in making lasting change. These include (but aren't limited to):

- **Positive psychology**, which leverages people's strengths (rather than focusing on their weaknesses) to make changes.
- **Motivational interviewing**, which helps people link behavior changes to their deepest needs and goals (e.g., "I will change my diet because I want to live to see my grandchildren graduate from college.").
- **Habit formation and reversal**, which supports patients in making positive habits, or breaking negative ones.

Each of these disciplines is supported by significant research. For example, a recent paper called "Effects of Positive Psychology Interventions on Risk Biomarkers in Coronary Patients" found that a positive psychology intervention lowered levels of C-reactive protein, an inflammatory marker, in patients with heart disease (Nikrahan et al. 2016). Another paper found that motivational interviewing increased the efficacy of a weight loss program in a group of overweight and obese women (Mirkarimi et al. 2015). Some research has shown that applying evidence-based principles of behavior change can increase the chances of success by over 1,000 percent (Grenny et al. 2008)!

Coaches are trained to work with patients in a more collaborative way, rather than with the expert approach that is common in medicine. In the expert approach, the "authority" assesses the problem, delivers advice, recommends solutions, and in some cases, teaches new skills. In the collaborative approach, the coach acts as a partner or ally, encourages the client to discover their own solutions and become their own advocate, and supports them in developing the skills they need to embrace new behaviors.

This collaborative approach empowers the client to become the primary driver of change. It also builds confidence, self-awareness, and self-actuation—all of which are crucial for long-term change, since the client will likely not work with the coach for the duration of his or her lifetime. To use an analogy, the doctor gives the patient a fish so she can eat for a day, whereas the coach teaches the client to fish so she can eat for a lifetime.

This more collaborative approach is also evidence-based: studies have consistently shown that coaching interventions improve health outcomes for several chronic diseases, including obesity (Appel et al. 2011), diabetes, heart disease, and cancer (Butterworth et al. 2006).

Anecdotal Evidence: The Importance of Clinical Experience

Another valuable trove of data comes from the anecdotal evidence doctors collect from working with patients. Anecdotal evidence is not reliable on its own, but it shouldn't be dismissed outright. Case studies can prompt new hypotheses and testing. Even when a treatment shines in a randomized clinical trial, it may be problematic in practice. Many patients experience side effects that people in the original study didn't—perhaps because there was a fluke in the research process or maybe because the side effects weren't reported. Evidence collected by interacting with patients is invaluable: it relates to real patients having real symptoms and can confirm or question the original research.

I might introduce a patient to a new treatment that looks

promising in the literature and watch carefully for neutral or negative results. If it doesn't work, or causes side effects, I'll revise my assessment of that treatment's efficacy and change my patients' recommendations accordingly. For example, several studies suggest that colostrum can be beneficial for a wide range of GI conditions, but my patients haven't experienced much success with it. That doesn't mean that it's not useful—perhaps other clinicians or another set of patients would experience greater success—but my anecdotal experience would lead me to pursue other options with my patient population.

"Evidence-based research" turns out to be more of a loaded term than we may have initially guessed.

PART FOUR

THE VISION

CHAPTER TWELVE

ADAPT IN PRACTICE: FOUR COMMON CONDITIONS

At its heart, the ADAPT Framework offers clinicians the opportunity to provide true healing, not merely temporary solutions. Most commonly prescribed drugs are just palliative—in other words, they offer some relief for symptoms but don't address the underlying cause (see table).

Medication	Primary Indication	Cures Underlying Problem?	Patient takes for life?
Synthroid	Hypothyroidism	No	Yes
Crestor	High cholesterol	No	Yes
Ventolin HFA	Asthma	No	Yes
Nexium	GERD	No	Yes
Advair Diskus	Asthma	No	Yes
Lantus Solostar	Diabetes	No	Yes
Vyvanse	ADHD	No	Yes
Lyrica	Pain/Fibromyalgia	No	Yes
Spiriva	Asthma, COPD	No	Yes
Januvia	Diabetes	No	Yes

Indications and usage of top 10 most prescribed drugs in the U.S. (Brown 2015)

What if practitioners could genuinely offer people the chance to reverse or even prevent chronic conditions, primarily through diet and lifestyle change, and occasionally supplements or other natural treatments? A practice like that would produce a myriad of positive results: reducing side effects, providing hope for patients who often don't have it, saving money over the long-term, dramatically improving quality of life, and providing a sense of empowerment for patients by putting them in charge of their own health and taking meaningful steps to improve it.

Let's compare how the ADAPT Framework differs from the conventional approach using four of the most commonly prescribed medications, and the conditions those medications are designed to treat.

Statins

Let's consider statins. Prescribing these drugs is typically the first step in conventional treatment of heart disease. In the Functional Medicine approach, we would look first at diet and lifestyle because that's the primary cause of dyslipidemia and hypercholesterolemia. After evaluating the patient's diet, we consider her physical activity, examine her sleep and stress management, and inspect her exposure to toxins—all areas that can affect lipoprotein and cholesterol levels.

Keeping the Exposome in mind, we remember that an ancestral diet and lifestyle will make a tremendous impact on this patient's cardiac health. Traditional populations, living closer to a hunter-gatherer diet and lifestyle, don't typically have high cholesterol or dyslipidemia, nor do they have any objective evidence of atherosclerosis (remember the Tsimané?). They're not taking statins, and they're not dying of heart attacks either. Therefore, we tackle diet and lifestyle first, recognizing that healthy change in these areas will make a profound difference as we move to subsequent steps.

Testing comes next, to identify any pathologies or underlying mechanisms that might be contributing to high cholesterol. We might test for poor thyroid function, which has been known for some time to impact cholesterol. We would also look at gut issues, like intestinal permeability ("leaky gut") or disrupted gut microbiome, as those also can contribute to high cholesterol. Then we'd move to examining metabolic issues like insulin or leptin resistance, which is common with diabetes. We might also look at exposure to heavy metals like lead and mercury and infections like *Helicobacter pylori*. These problems can all lead to high cholesterol and a high LDL particle number (Kresser 2013b; Asgary et al. 2017). After testing, we would do specific treatments to address those issues.

To be fair, although most conventional practitioners are not testing for these underlying causes, it's likely that many would at least encourage diet and lifestyle changes. At that point in a conventional model, the doctor would simply issue his or her recommendations: "Okay, eat better. Exercise more. Do this protocol." The patient would walk away and then likely struggle or fail to follow through. But in the ADAPT Framework, we use allied providers like nurse practitioners, physician assistants, health coaches, and nutritionists, all of whom can help the patient implement the clinician's recommendations. This collaboration among team members—a team that includes the patient—is far more likely to ensure the patient makes the necessary changes to improve his or her long-term health.

DIET VS. DRUGS

In his book, *Catastrophic Care*, David Goldhill remarked: "Before the invention of statins, [a cardiac patient] would have needed a change of diet to reduce the risk of heart disease. The invention of statins provided not only a medical alternative, but an alternative that others, through insurance, would help me pay for." (Goldhill 2013, 103.)

Goldhill is arguing that his cardiologist told him he needed to eat more fish, fruits, and vegetables, and less ice cream, burgers, and donuts—or, just take a statin. The implication is that these two approaches are equivalent, as if a statin will have the same impact of not eating donuts and ice cream. This exemplifies the natural consequences of a system that puts most of its emphasis on drugs.

Patients conclude, "Well, if my doctor isn't taking time to emphasize diet and lifestyle, then this drug must be an alternative. Taking the drug is easier, and my insurance pays for it. Insurance isn't going to pay for new groceries or a gym membership, though—plus, changing my diet and lifestyle sounds like a lot of work." Yet patients need to recognize that the system is set up to support and subsidize drugs— its mode of intervention is superficial. When patients grow accustomed to being passive recipients of care, rather than being actively engaged in their own lifestyle changes, symptomatic problems will persist, and root cause healing will elude them.

Bronchodilators

Albuterol, used for asthma, is the third most prescribed medication in the United States (Brown 2015). The conventional narrative that accompanies an asthma diagnosis is this: "You have difficulty breathing, so carry around this inhaler and use it whenever an attack starts up. That's what you'll want to do for the rest of your life. Good luck!" Many people have heard some version of this diagnosis. Asthma is a huge problem, affecting almost 10 percent of the population—25 million Americans—a number that increases every day (CDC 2011).

How would we approach an asthmatic patient in the ADAPT Framework? Many aspects of the modern diet and lifestyle have been identified as contributors to asthma, such as processed and refined food, sensitivities to food additives and dyes, and environmental toxins (especially airborne toxins). Research has found that a sedentary lifestyle, chronic stress, and sleep deprivation can all be contributing factors, too. Our modern diet and lifestyle—so clearly mismatched to how humans were made to function—make this problem more common.

Our functional model would then lead us to look for the pathologies behind the asthma, especially gut dysfunction. The modern lifestyle has disrupted the gut microbiome, causing intestinal permeability and increases in food sensitivity, all of which contribute to asthma. We would look at nutrient status with blood testing, examine hormone levels, and check vitamin D levels. We would do extensive testing to find the contributing underlying mechanisms and address each one as they were discovered.

Like the high cholesterol and statin example, the ADAPT Framework would then set up this asthmatic patient with allied providers and a higher-touch level of care, so that the patient had the support needed to make these meaningful changes.

Antidepressants

Abilify, the anti-psychotic medication we touched on briefly in Chapter Eleven, is also worth examining as a case study on how Functional Medicine approaches illness differently. To recap: on-label, Abilify is used to treat schizophrenia, bipolar disorder, and Tourette's syndrome. It's also being used off-label to treat depression and is even being used with children to treat irritability associated with autism spectrum disorder.

Let's look more closely at how drugs like this came to be accepted as treatments for disorders like depression. Early research on depression suggested that it stems from an imbalance in brain chemistry; some people are susceptible and others are not. If a patient has low serotonin levels in the brain, the thinking went, they can take a drug that boosts serotonin availability. Then, they continue taking the drug for the rest of their lives.

Many of the assumptions made in this scenario turned out to be problematic. Research suggests that depression is not actually caused by low serotonin (Cowen and Browning 2015). Large reviews have shown that serotonin-based antidepressants may not be any more effective than placebos, at least for mild to moderate depression (Fournier et al. 2010). Even more concerning from a Functional Medicine perspective, the drugs don't address the underlying causes of depression in a curative way.

One of the most recent theories about potential causes of depression is called the "Immune Cytokine Model of Depression" (Smith 2010; Kresser 2016). This theory holds that inflammation, often originating in the gut, produces chemical messengers called cytokines. These cytokines then travel through the blood stream, cross the blood brain barrier, and suppress the activity of the frontal cortex. That, in turn, causes the symptoms that we label as depression. If that's the case, then the solution to depression is not to increase serotonin availability in the brain, but to reduce inflammation, particularly in the gut.

Once again, we start with the Exposome, looking at any diet, behavior, or lifestyle triggers that would cause inflammation. Certainly, there are many triggers to be found in our inflammatory highly processed and refined diet. Other culprits might be a sedentary lifestyle, shallow sleep, poor stress management, a lack of social support, and/or exposure to environmental toxins that provoke an inflammatory response. We would systematically identify and address all diet, lifestyle, and behavior factors that contribute to inflammation.

From a Functional Medicine perspective, we would, of course, do a thorough work-up to determine any other hidden causes of inflammation, such as parasite infection, disrupted gut microbiome, and intestinal permeability. We would look at HPA access dysregulation (problems with cortisol and stress-related pathology), which is known to be a trigger for inflammation. We would look at nutrient balance, checking for deficiencies of iron, magnesium, B-vitamins, and vitamin D, or an excess such as iron overload. Blood sugar issues would be examined, as high blood sugar can contribute to an inflammatory response. We would also look for things like mold and biotoxin exposure, and chronic infections. There are several underlying pathologies that provoke inflammation. We would look at them all.

The high touch aspect of the ADAPT model is especially

important for a patient working through a psychological ailment. In a higher-touch practice model, the doctor has more time to spend with the patient and truly get a sense of what other factors might be contributing to depression—both from a diet, lifestyle, and behavior perspective, and from a psychological and emotional perspective. The support from staff allied providers can remind the patient he or she is not alone in making lifestyle changes.

Stimulants

Behavioral disorders like ADHD are becoming increasingly common, especially in children. The CDC estimates that 11 percent of children four to seventeen years of age have been diagnosed with ADHD, and that diagnoses have increased by 42 percent in the last eight years (CDC 2017a).

The conventional approach to treating ADHD typically involves prescribing a stimulant drug such as Vyvanse (which explains why it is the seventh most frequently prescribed drug in the United States). Although these medications can be helpful in controlling the symptoms, they do not address the underlying cause of the problem.

What might these causes be? If you look up ADHD on mainstream health websites, they will tell you that the causes of ADHD are unknown. They mention that some genetic predispositions have been identified, but otherwise we don't know. Some sources even go out of their way to suggest that diet has not been shown to have any effect on ADHD.

If you look in the scientific literature, however, and consider ADHD from a Functional Medicine perspective, you'll find that there are several compelling theories for what causes it and why it has increased so significantly over the past several years. One such theory is known as the "Three Hit Paradigm," in which three key influences—or "hits"—combine and contribute to not only ADHD but other behavioral conditions in both children and adults (Slattery et al. 2016). The three hits are:

1. **Biome depletion:** this refers to the depletion of the microbiome due to poor diet, overuse of antibiotics, and other aspects of the modern lifestyle.
2. **Environmental stimulus at critical times in development:** e.g. acetaminophen exposure, vitamin D deficiency, antibiotic exposure, and other diet and lifestyle influences.
3. **Genetic and/or epigenetic predisposition.**

With this perspective, we can examine a wide range of potential underlying causes, including poor diet, nutrient deficiency, exposure to toxins (including pharmaceutical drugs like acetaminophen that can have a toxic effect), poor folate metabolism or absorption, and gut health. Then, we can address each of these causes and significantly improve or even completely reverse the condition, instead of just suppressing symptoms with drugs.

The differences between these approaches have a profound impact on both the children suffering from these conditions and their parents. The conventional approach offers little hope for true healing; it simply suggests that the child has a deficiency of some kind that can only be managed by a lifetime of medication use. On the other hand, the Functional Medicine approach offers the possibility of real transformation. It provides an explanation for why the child is suffering from these problems, one that recognizes the many external factors that have contributed to the attention deficit behaviors. And with that, it enables the parents, the child, and the healthcare provider to work together to address these causes and promote meaningful and lasting change.

CHAPTER THIRTEEN

ADAPT IN PRACTICE: THE PRACTITIONER'S EXPERIENCE

In Chapter Ten, we examined several differences between a conventional medical practice, and a collaborative practice model. In this chapter, we'll dive more deeply into the practitioner's experience of the ADAPT Framework.

The Clinician's Experience

Let's explore a day in the life of a clinician—we'll call her Anjali—who has recently made the transition from conventional medicine to practicing Functional Medicine within the ADAPT Framework.

Looking forward to the day

Like many other physicians, Anjali was feeling burned out and drained in her conventional practice. The days were long, and she never felt that she truly helped her patients. After several years of this, she began to wake up on work days with a sense of dread. This was especially hard for her since she is naturally an optimistic person with a positive attitude.

But this morning, as Anjali prepares for her day, she can hardly wait to get started. She's excited because she knows she'll be able to offer her patients real solutions to their problems, rather than just suppressing symptoms with drugs. On a typical day in her conventional practice, she might have seen up to twenty-five patients; today, she has only eight visits scheduled: three new patients, and five established patients.

Plenty of time to prepare

Because of this lighter schedule, Anjali has plenty of time to prepare for her new patients. Her appointments don't begin until 10:00 a.m., so she sits down with a cup of coffee in her home office and reviews the intake paper-work and lab tests for each of her new patients. As she reads each patient's detailed medical history and examines their test results, she creates a report of her findings, which lists the underlying pathologies she believes are contributing to the patient's complaints, makes recommendations for further testing, and outlines the treatment plan. Once she completes these reports, she feels much more confident about her approach; when she walks into the room with them, she'll be prepared with not only a thorough understanding of their case but a comprehensive plan for addressing their problems. This is a dramatic change from her previous practice, where she rushed from one appointment to the next, always feeling like she was just skimming the surface and offering Band-Aids rather than real solutions.

A better work environment

When Anjali opens the front door, and enters the waiting room of her office, she smiles to herself. Instead of the harsh fluorescent lights, sterile white walls, and harried vibe she encountered in her previous practice, Anjali's new office is beautiful, peaceful, and relaxing. It's infused with natural light, with earth-toned walls, tasteful and comfortable furniture, and a small fountain in the corner. She heads back to the small kitchen to make herself a cup of tea, before entering her consultation room. This room has wood floors, a window facing a garden, a desk for her to sit at, and a sofa for her patients. It has soft halogen lighting, several plants, and tasteful artwork on the walls. Anjali opens her laptop and reviews the documents she prepared earlier for a few minutes before her first patient arrives.

Solving problems and offering hope

Anjali's first patient, Maya, has severe rosacea that hasn't responded to conventional treatment. Maya had seen several dermatologists, including the chair of the dermatology department at the local medical school. She'd tried topical antibiotics, sulfa-based face washes, and even isotretinoin, a medication with potentially serious side effects. None made a significant difference. During Anjali's review of Maya's labs, she discovers that Maya has severe SIBO. Anjali knows that this is a key finding, since she had recently read a study indicating that SIBO is common in patients with acne rosacea, and that treating it leads to either complete resolution or significant improvement in most cases (Butterworth et al. 2006). Anjali prescribed a botanical treatment for SIBO that has been shown in studies to be as effective as the pharmaceutical treatment, with fewer side effects and risks. For the first time in many years and numerous visits to the doctor, Maya left feeling hopeful and encouraged that she finally had a solution to her skin problem.

Anjali's next patient, Aidan, is a fifty-eight-year-old male complaining of brain fog, memory loss, difficulty with word recall, and decreased cognitive function. Aidan is VP of business development of a technology company, and he's alarmed by the decline in his ability to think clearly, retain information, and perform at work. Aidan's PCP referred him to a neurologist, who ran some tests and told him that his genes predisposed him to a higher risk of dementia and Alzheimer's and that these symptoms may reflect the onset of those conditions. This didn't sit well with Aidan because his symptoms had started rather abruptly after he moved into a new home about six months ago. Anjali had also noticed the timing of the onset of Aidan's symptoms in her detailed review of his history. What's more, Aidan indicated that he noticed musty smells in this house, and that the crawl space has visible mold growing on the walls. A few months before this appointment, Anjali attended a seminar with Dr. Dale Bredesen (whom we met earlier in the book), where she learned about a type of dementia and Alzheimer's disease that is caused by exposure to toxins like heavy metals and mold. Anjali had included some biomarkers for this in the initial testing she ordered for Aidan, and several of them came back positive. Anjali explains to

Aidan that his symptoms may be related to exposure to mold in his new home. She recommends a reputable mold assessment company locally that can test Aidan's house and make recommendations for remediation. She also prescribes treatment to support healthy detoxification, reduce inflammation, and restore cognitive function. Aidan leaves Anjali's office feeling empowered and optimistic. After his visit to the neurologist, he felt hopeless as he contemplated the inexorable decline in mental health that he knew happened in dementia and Alzheimer's patients. But now he not only had an explanation for his symptoms that made sense to him, he had several steps he could take to reverse those symptoms.

Anjali's third patient is an eight-year-old boy named Tyler, who suffers from a long list of allergies (to both foods and environmental antigens like dust and pollen), asthma, and frequent colds and flus. Tyler's parents had consulted with his pediatrician, an immunologist, and a pulmonologist. Not surprisingly, these practitioners prescribed several medications. Some of the drugs were at least mildly helpful, but none made a significant difference in Tyler's condition. Tyler's mother discovered Functional Medicine in her online research about his condition, and she was immediately drawn to it. Although Tyler's issues are not uncommon among kids today, his mom always felt that there must be a *reason* for this: she intuitively knew that it's not normal for kids to have such compromised immune function. Anjali ran a similar panel of tests that she had used with her adult patients, Aidan and Maya. She found that Tyler had a severely disrupted gut microbiome, with low levels of beneficial microbes and high levels of pathogenic bacteria and yeast. Anjali was not surprised by this because in Tyler's intake paperwork his mom noted that he was born via cesarean section and was not breast-fed—both factors that are associated with a disrupted gut microbiome. Anjali also found that Tyler was deficient in several nutrients critical to proper immune function, including magnesium, zinc, selenium, vitamin C, and vitamin D. Finally, Tyler tested positive for intolerance to gluten and dairy, foods that he was still eating because the immunologist they consulted said that Tyler wasn't allergic to them. Anjali explained to Tyler's mom that intolerance and allergy are not the same thing, and that although allergy typically produces a more serious (and sometimes even life-threatening response), intolerance can also provoke significant symptoms, including immune dysregulation. Anjali prescribes an ancestral diet that is strictly gluten- and dairy-free, botanicals and supplements to reduce the pathogens in Tyler's gut, probiotics and prebiotics to increase his beneficial bacteria, and some supplements to improve his nutrient status. Tyler's mom leaves the appointment feeling relieved that she's finally found some answers, and hopeful that this new plan will enable Tyler to get off his medications and begin to truly heal.

A collaborative model with more support for patients

As Anjali finishes her last new patient appointment for the day and heads across the street for lunch, she reflects on how different her experience as a doctor is now. Three years ago, if these patients had come to see her when she was working in the conventional model, she would have had little to offer them other than a prescription for a drug. She wouldn't have had the time to do a thorough intake and review of the patients' history; insurance restrictions would have prevented her from ordering the lab tests that were instrumental in her diagnoses; and even if she had been able to correctly diagnose the problems, she wouldn't have had the training to treat them effectively or the infrastructure to support patients in making the necessary changes.

Fortunately, in her new practice, Anjali has both the knowledge to treat these conditions as well as the freedom to prescribe the interventions she thinks would be most helpful (rather than being tied to those that the insurance company has decided to reimburse). Moreover, she has a nurse practitioner and a health coach (who is also a nutritionist) on staff who can provide an additional layer of support for her patients. This turns out to be especially helpful in Tyler's case; he has two brothers and a sister, so his parents have a lot on their plate and they are feeling overwhelmed by the magnitude of the changes Anjali is asking them to make. The health coach will be able to work closely with Tyler's parents, giving them handouts that walk them through the supplement protocols, making suggestions for healthy foods that Tyler will eat on his new diet, providing recipes and meal plans, and offering moral support when needed. The nurse practitioner will also be available to help answer any follow-up questions related to the treatment protocol, address any side effects that Tyler may experience, and adjust dosages or change supplements as necessary.

The support of the health coach and nurse practitioner is not only a game-changer for Anjali's patients, it also dramatically improves her experience as a clinician. Her patients are far more likely to follow through with her recommendations, which in turn leads to much more successful outcomes. And since Anjali doesn't need to provide this support herself, she is able to maintain a manageable schedule while still offering a very high level of service to her patients. In fact, since she hired the health coach and NP, Anjali has been able to drop a full day of clinic time each week, which she has used for research and continuing education, spending more time with her family, and beginning to realize her long-time dream of learning to play the piano.

Streamlined operations and more time with patients

After lunch, Anjali walks back to the office to prepare for the afternoon's appointments. She has five visits with existing patients; two forty-five-minute appointments, and three thirty-minute appointments. Three of the visits are in the office, and two are virtual via a HIPAA-compliant videoconferencing platform.

By this point in her day in her previous job, Anjali was already feeling exhausted. She went from one brief appointment to the next, with hardly enough time to say hello to patients, much less do a thorough review of their symptoms, lab tests, and treatment protocol and explore their diet, lifestyle, and behavior. Anjali's prior employer did use an electronic health record (EHR), but it was plagued with problems and rather than speeding up workflow and providing more time with patients, it always seemed to have the opposite effect.

In her new practice, Anjali is using a different EHR that is optimized for Functional Medicine and the ADAPT practice model. All of Anjali's established patients fill out a progress update form prior to their visit, which asks them to list any medications and supplements they're taking; to rate their overall health on a scale of 1-10; rate symptoms like energy, pain, and cognitive function since their last appointment on a scale of 1-5, with one being worse, and five being better; document any significant changes or updates since their last appointment; and list the three most important issues or questions they want to discuss during the appointment, as well as other concerns they'd like to cover if time allows.

Anjali's EHR also allows her to quickly access the appointment notes from any visits with the health coach or nurse practitioner that Anjali's patients may have had between appointments with her. This makes it easy for Anjali to stay informed about her patients' progress and provides important continuity of care.

Independence and autonomy

As Anjali moves through her afternoon visits, she is free to make recommendations and prescribe treatments she thinks are best in each situation, based on her research and ongoing study. That wasn't the case in her previous practice where she was bound by standard of care and limited to the treatments that the insurance company would pay for (what I referred to as "reimbursement-based medicine" earlier in Chapter Three). Anjali knows that many of the newest scientific discoveries related to diagnosis and treatment take years, if not decades, to be adopted by insurance companies and primary care groups. She is grateful that in her new practice she has not only the time to do research and stay abreast of the latest developments but also the freedom and autonomy to order these new evidence-based tests and treatments for her patients.

For example, one of Anjali's afternoon patients has Crohn's disease. The typical treatments—and the ones insurance companies will pay for—are steroids like prednisone, aminosalicylates like mesalamine, or biologics like infliximab. While these medications can be helpful in reducing inflammation, and are sometimes necessary, they do not address the underlying cause of the problem: autoimmunity. They also have significant side effects and risks, especially in the case of steroids and biologics. Anjali used a different approach with this patient that involved an antimicrobial protocol to treat a previously undiagnosed gut infection, a special diet to reduce inflammation in the GI tract, and a low-dose of a medication called naltrexone, which is used at full dose to assist with opioid withdrawal, but has recently been shown to regulate the immune system and even induce remission in patients with autoimmune disease at lower doses. She is happy to hear that her patient is doing well and has not needed to take any of her previous medications, which included prednisone and mesalamine. In her previous practice, Anjali would not have had the autonomy, time, or support she needed to use this more holistic protocol.

Meaning, purpose, and passion

The differences I mentioned above between Anjali's conventional practice and her current ADAPT Framework-inspired practice are so dramatic that her experience at work is almost unrecognizable to her. Whereas before she felt a sense of dread at the beginning of the day, and exhaustion before she had even made it to the end of the day, now Anjali literally jumps out of bed with excitement. Like Sherry, the clinician we met in Chapter Six, Anjali was considering a career change prior to discovering this new approach; she simply couldn't imagine another decade of conventional medical practice. It had taken a huge toll on her health. She had gained weight, was starting to show early signs of diabetes, was having trouble sleeping, and didn't have any energy left over for her husband and kids in the evenings or on the weekends.

But perhaps the biggest and most important difference for Anjali has been the strong sense of meaning and purpose that she now feels in her work. Like many physicians, Anjali chose medicine because she truly wanted to help people. As a young child, she displayed unusual empathy and concern for other people, and she entered medical school feeling idealistic and inspired to make a difference in her patient's lives. But even before she finished medical school, this clear sense of purpose had become a vague memory. The reality of her residency—short appointments, an almost exclusive focus on pharmacotherapy, and little time to form meaningful relationships with patients—turned out to be far different than her dreams of what being a doctor would be like.

Fortunately for Anjali, through Functional Medicine and the ADAPT Framework, she discovered a way of practicing medicine that restored her lifelong sense of purpose: to be a healer who truly transforms her patients' lives. She has a renewed passion for her work and cannot imagine retiring because it feeds her so deeply. This is the potential of this approach for all healthcare practitioners.

The Allied Provider's Experience

The ADAPT Framework offers physicians the opportunity to help patients achieve lasting, curative healing. Patients, likewise, are freed from chronic illness and buoyed by the support of a collaborative healthcare team.

But what about the other members of that team? What does it offer the nurse practitioners, physician assistants, coaches, and nutritionists who are also participating in the patient's healing?

ADAPT offers allied providers a methodology and a framework. In many other contexts, allied providers find themselves in a situation where they don't know where to start, or how to structure and layer an intervention with patients. They might recommend a diet change here, or supplement there, or lifestyle change there, but it's not systematic. It's not based in a framework or methodology, or even a narrative that makes sense to the patient or the client.

Allied providers trained in the ADAPT Framework have an immediate place to start in providing a narrative to the patient. When allied providers explain the mismatch concept and importance of an ancestral diet and life-style to patients, they offer a firm rationale that puts the changes they're making into a larger context. Having this context empowers patients to identify other areas of their lives where there may be a mismatch. Simply having that framework supports the changes; patients start to see their lives and choices from a different perspective. Certain behaviors or diet choices or lifestyle choices may have seemed normal because it's all they've ever known, but now they begin to see that those choices are not "normal," even though they're common. Those choices contribute to their health problems. With the help of their support team, patients realize they can take meaningful steps toward better choices. They learn why they need to change, what they need to change, and how to make those changes.

Licensed allied providers—such as nurse practitioners and physician assistants—are also given the Functional Medicine tool set, to be able to diagnose and identify underlying causes of disease. Suddenly, these providers can do more than just suppress symptoms, ultimately making them far more effective at their jobs. As the doctor shortage worsens, allied providers are going to be increasingly on the front lines in ordering tests and prescribing care. They are the ones interfacing most often with patients, and do most of the legwork. Training in the functional approach and methodology is crucial for their ability to help their patients.

It's also important for the non-licensed providers—like nutritionists and health coaches—to understand the core principles of Functional Medicine, even if they're not ordering tests and writing prescriptions. The fundamental paradigm of practicing root cause medicine, understanding that diet, lifestyle, and behavior are at the root of all chronic disease, is tremendously empowering for non-licensed allied providers. Seeing healthcare this way reminds them they're the most important link in the chain. These non-licensed providers work intensively with clients to accomplish the most necessary changes in their treatment.

Like patients, non-licensed providers need a support team. Too often now, nutritionists and health coaches have no regular way to communicate with the licensed providers in their practice. When a patient appears at their door, they may not know about medications the doctor has prescribed. Similarly, when the patient returns to the doctor, he or she might not mention the supplements the health coach recommended. What if the medication and the supplements are at odds? That's problematic for everyone involved.

The ADAPT model advocates frequent communication and a close working relationship. In this model, allied providers experience more respect and likely more consistent work because they receive frequent referrals from the licensed provider. Some allied providers might get to experience working inside a collaborative clinic environment with other providers, receiving a salary and benefits. Many health coaches and nutritionists feel isolated at times because they work independently coaching clients; they miss the collaborative process of bouncing ideas off other colleagues. The ADAPT model advocates for close collaboration within a team of physicians and allied providers, recognizing all the advantages that come from doing so.

CHAPTER FOURTEEN

ADAPT IN PRACTICE: THE PATIENT'S EXPERIENCE

In the last chapter, we saw how practicing within the ADAPT Framework—especially after working in a conventional setting—can be enormously freeing for the practitioner. The same holds true for the patient but perhaps even more so. Let's spend some time with patients to see how the two worlds look to them.

First Impressions

Functional Medicine clinics try to create an environment that feels conducive to health and healing. As I mentioned in the last chapter, that might include soft lighting, tasteful décor, and a peaceful, quiet space with comfortable seating. It might strike a patient more as a massage therapy office or spa than a typical doctor's office.

A patient might feel surprised by this initial impression; he's probably used to harsh fluorescent lighting and busy waiting rooms. Often, the staff in conventional offices seems to be harried and stressed. Most of the patient's past office visits probably took place in rooms with white walls and white ceilings; the environment typically felt sterile and a bit cold.

Plenty of Time With Doctor

After being invited into an appointment, the patient at a Functional Medicine practice leaves the restful waiting room to sit down with the clinician. The patient—let's call him Jerome—is accustomed to feeling nervous in this moment. In past appointments, Jerome typically felt anxious as he wondered how he could describe everything that he wanted to talk about in the short time allotted. Now, there's plenty of time for thorough conversation. He feels relieved. The clinician invites him into his office, which has a desk, a chair, and sometimes a couch. There may be a table set up to accommodate a physical exam, if necessary. Once again, Jerome is surprised; this office feels like a therapy office, not a sterile clinic.

Active vs. Passive Role

During the appointment, the clinician encourages Jerome to play an active role in his experience. The clinician begins by inviting Jerome's opinions. What does he think is going on? Jerome may wonder why nobody's ever asked him these questions before. He remembers one or two former doctors who encouraged him to express himself, but usually he just feels intimidated and clams up. He did once mention a treatment he had read about online to his PCP, and asked his doctor if he thought it might help, but the idea was quickly dismissed as amateur. After that, Jerome didn't voice his ideas anymore. He didn't want to expose his ignorance—not when his doctor seemed to know so much more than he did.

And yet, his symptoms remained. The prescriptions from his PCP hadn't helped, so he kept researching on his own. Finally, he stumbled across information about ancestral health and Functional Medicine. He cut out processed foods and sugar, and reduced his intake of grains and dairy. This seemed to help. But when he returned to his doctor and ventured a question about Functional Medicine, the PCP was once again dismissive. "That's not real medicine. But if you feel like you need further treatment, let's set you up with a specialist."

So Jerome went to the specialists. Maybe they would have

the solution. If doctors were the experts, then surely specialists would be the very gatekeepers of information. But even the specialists let him down. Years after starting his pursuit of better health, after taking multiple prescriptions and keeping countless appointments, Jerome's symptoms weren't any better.

Eventually, Jerome finds himself in a Functional Medicine clinic, sitting on a couch, facing a very different kind of doctor. The intake form had been like nothing he'd ever completed—the questions were about far more than medical history or symptoms. They had asked about his profession and his interests, his past experiences with medical care, and what he was looking for in a healthcare practitioner. One question had asked, "What is your opinion on what has happened to your health?" The first thought that occurs to Jerome is: "I can't believe my doctor wants to hear my opinion."

Yet this is exactly what a Functional Medicine clinician wants to hear: we know that the key changes are going to come from the patients, so we're eager to hear the patient's input and ideas. Functional Medicine doesn't work if the patient doesn't actively participate in changing his behavior, diet, and lifestyle. We don't want patients to feel like mere medication recipients. We want their motivated participation. In fact, one question on our clinic's intake form asks patients to measure their motivation: "On a scale of one to ten, how committed are you to recovering your health?" We get the best results with highly motivated and committed patients who can apply our recommendations, so this is useful information.

Jerome may be wondering by now what's going on. He had expected a brief consultation and a new sort of pill. Instead, this new doctor tells him he's going to be expected to play a participatory role. He was used to operating under the assumption that pills alone would solve his problems. That might be true if he had an acute infectious disease, but he's dealing with a chronic illness that requires a different kind of treatment. As they talk, Jerome realizes he now has a very different role as a patient.

Jerome's practitioner explains the necessary shift: "Our typical modern lifestyle is at odds with our genes and biology, and that's what's causing your symptoms. But if you can bring your diet and lifestyle more in alignment with what we know is appropriate for us as a species, you have greater potential to address your complaints than any pill does." By the end of the session, Jerome has learned about a system for implementing those changes and received referrals to a support team to help him do it.

Taking Responsibility for One's Own Health

Over the course of his appointment, Jerome starts feeling empowered. The power to heal no longer rested solely in the doctor's hands. He didn't have to follow blindly along, taking exactly what they told him to take, without question. Now he is the primary agent in his own care. With this realization comes a new hope and a sense of validation he may not have known he was missing. Jerome had started to worry that his symptoms were a result of his own personal problems, a failure of willpower. Now he understands that chronic illness might be more a result of environmental and cultural factors. Perhaps his problems don't stem from any personal lack but are a result of sitting at a desk for eight hours a day. Maybe it has something to do with his exposure to blue light while he watches movies on his iPad before bed. Could that be what's keeping him awake at night?

As the Functional Medicine patient's gaze turns from an inner sense of failure to an outward view of empowered action, he starts to think about the areas of his life that are inconsistent with his natural human template. If he can identify those, he can choose positive lifestyle changes.

He also is now better equipped to make those changes. Conventional diet plans are notoriously difficult to maintain. They may be hard to follow or unappetizing. The recommendations given to him by his new doctor, based on an ancestral diet, are somehow more satisfying. He's not hungry all the time! What's happening here? When Jerome asks this in a follow-up appointment, his doctor explains that the diet is geared to meet human genetic requirements, and therefore does a better job answering our cravings than other diets. Because the patient feels more satisfied with this way of eating, he can continue consistently and happily.

Jerome makes other lifestyle changes as well. Although he's heard some of this advice before, it feels more doable with an evolutionary framework guiding him. Jerome knew he should get more exercise but after sitting at his desk for eight hours, the last thing he wanted to do was head to the gym for an hour and run on a treadmill, as a previous doctor advised. In this case, his Functional Medicine doctor helps him brainstorm ways to avoid sitting all day. "The point is not just to get exercise but also increase your non-exercise physical activity all around," his doctor urges. Jerome develops a mixed routine where he's standing and walking at work and sitting less. Moving more throughout the day gives him more energy to pursue high intensity activities outside of work. It's easier to maintain consistency—especially with the check-ins from the Functional Medicine clinic—and he feels noticeably better. As a result, the new routine sticks.

Jerome finally feels like he has someone on his side. He has honestly connected with his doctor after many generous appointments filled with respectful conversations. His doctor's advocacy and the support of a coach and allied providers make a profound difference in his determination to participate in his healing.

Allied Provider Interactions

Those allied providers are an important part of a patient's experience in the Functional Medicine model. Let's say a patient named Kevin comes to our clinic with rheumatoid arthritis, an autoimmune disease. The initial consult takes place with the nurse practitioner. Kevin senses he's speaking to a professional who understands his situation and trusts she will perform a thorough and informed interview to ensure the right information is collected for determining a successful treatment.

Kevin then goes on to have his case review with the clinician. The clinician goes over the patient's data, forms, and paperwork and prescribes a treatment plan. Especially given this patient's autoimmune disease, the treatment plan might be extensive. It might involve an autoimmune diet protocol and could require some herbs and supplements to address Kevin's gut issues. The clinician will likely want Kevin to focus on stress management because stress is a big factor in autoimmune disease. There might also be a focus on appropriate physical activity and movement because that's important for arthritic conditions.

That's quite a list. Even if Kevin is highly motivated to make these changes, he might still feel overwhelmed by the complexity of his treatment. Left to his own devices, he's going to have a difficult time carrying them all out successfully. Enter: the health coach. The coach provides resources like handouts that describe the diet protocol in more detail. She answers any questions, and helps the patient gear up for his dietary changes, giving him practical advice about where to shop for new ingredients and how to prepare his food. She'll also provide information on stress management resources, like tools that can help monitor sleep. She outlines options for physical activity, and perhaps refers Kevin to a local physical trainer who has experience with rheumatoid arthritis clients. Or if the health coach is experienced herself, she can suggest some at-home exercises to try. As Kevin navigates the ups and downs of his treatment plan, he can regularly touch base with his coach. She will help him break the changes down into bite-sized pieces, perhaps suggesting which step to focus on first. With this support, he is far more likely to be successful with his treatment plan—and far more likely to start experiencing real improvement.

Technological Support

Kevin's experience at the Functional Medicine clinic is also supported through a variety of technological touchpoints. He can regularly log into a patient portal and communicate with his providers. He has immediate online access to all his lab reports and the handouts he's received. He can send a follow-up question to his clinician after an appointment and receive a response within forty-eight hours. This regular interaction with his providers feels efficient and effective, and the regular dialog helps him continue with his diet and lifestyle changes.

If the Functional Medicine practice Kevin visits also uses telemedicine, he can easily maintain consistent contact with his care team. If he must travel for a business conference, for example, he can still make his Wednesday appointment by video during his lunch break and continue his treatment on the optimal timetable.

Payment

So how much does all of this cost the patient? In Chapter Eight I explained that, although Functional Medicine will almost certainly prove more cost-effective than conventional medicine over time, right now out-of-pocket expenses are higher for Functional Medicine because of the lack of insurance coverage. Patients may have to increase the amount of money they initially invest in their health, understanding that, like with other good investments, they'll receive a significant return over time. Most find the investment in Functional Medicine to be worth it because they receive a high level of care that helps them address problems more effectively and consistently than ever before.

It's worth noting that conventional care can be enormously expensive for patients since it relies heavily on medications, surgery, and other expensive procedures. Insurance provides some relief but doesn't always cover these expenses—and when that happens the results can be disastrous. One in five Americans struggle to pay medical bills each year. Three in five bankruptcies are due to medical expenses, making health care the number one cause of such filings, even ahead of unpaid credit cards or mortgages (LaMontagne 2013).

Functional Medicine, with its emphasis on preventing and reversing disease rather than just suppressing symptoms with medication, can potentially save patients thousands of dollars over the course of their life. Latisha, the patient with Crohn's disease and diabetes that we met in Chapter Four, is a perfect example. She was forced to stop working and go on long-term disability, and eventually had to declare bankruptcy, because of her conditions. With a

Functional Medicine approach, she may have been able to reverse or at least control her Crohn's disease, and prevent the onset of type 2 diabetes. She could have kept her job and avoided the steady accumulation of unpaid medical bills that eventually bankrupted her. Functional Medicine, though more expensive initially, could have saved Latisha tens of thousands of dollars in direct medical costs over a lifetime—not to mention the tens or even hundreds of thousands of dollars she forfeited from lost income, savings, and investments. So, even without insurance coverage, in some cases Functional Medicine can be significantly cheaper than a conventional approach.

PART FIVE

THE
TRANSITION

CHAPTER FIFTEEN

THE FUTURE OF MEDICINE

By now, I hope I've convinced you that the ADAPT Framework is truly the future of medicine.

That future can't arrive soon enough. The healthcare debate in 2017 revealed, among other things, just how precarious our current system has become. No recent political issue has drawn more public comments and interest. When the Trump administration proposed changes to the Affordable Care Act that would result in millions of people losing coverage, and fewer benefits for those who do have coverage, politicians were overwhelmed with the response. During standing-room only town hall meetings, people across the U.S. shared how they would be affected by the proposed changes. A mother in tears described how her daughter, who had been diagnosed with leukemia, wouldn't be able to get the treatment she needed. A disabled man in a wheelchair who depends on Medicaid wondered how he'd survive without it. Hundreds of citizens across the U.S. expressed their anger, fear, and opposition to the proposed changes.

The Symptoms Are Clear, but the Diagnosis and Treatment Are Wrong

These stories are heartbreaking, and the needs they reveal are serious and demanding of attention and support. But the public discussion of these issues fell short in one crucial way: it correctly recognized the symptom (a failing healthcare system), but the diagnosis (not enough insurance coverage) and the prescription for solving it (more insurance coverage) were incomplete. Throughout the entire debate, neither politicians nor the media acknowledged the *real* reason that healthcare is doomed to fail in this country, nor did they propose a solution that was anything other than the equivalent of bailing water from a sinking boat.

Back in Chapter Four, I said:

Making a few small tweaks to our current system and

expecting that to work is like rearranging the deck furniture on the Titanic as it inexorably sinks into the ocean. Too little, too late.

If chronic disease continues to grow at the current pace, an insurance-based healthcare system is destined to fail. There's just no way to effectively pay for the care needed in a country this large, when one in two adults and one in four children have a chronic disease. This is the "dirty secret" that no one wants to acknowledge.

We have come to equate health with healthcare, but that is a fallacy. As David Goldhill explains in *Catastrophic Care*, "The factors that most predict your health are your wealth, education, and lifestyle—not your access to healthcare. These personal and societal investments are the real 'preventative' care, yet they are buried under our growing demand for tests and procedures." (Goldhill 2013, 26.)

Along the same lines, *health insurance isn't health care*. Health insurance is a *method for paying for health care*. Although it's the one we're most familiar with, it's relatively new. Private group insurance was introduced in 1929, employer-based insurance didn't take off until World War II, and as late as the mid-1950s only a minority of Americans had health insurance. At that time, Congress introduced legislation that made employer contributions to employee health plans tax deductible for businesses, and the number of people with health insurance grew exponentially. Goldhill again explains, "In short, a minor tax benefit passed more than half a century ago is the source of all of our cultural assumptions surrounding health care." (Goldhill 2013, 26.)

A Better Way

I'm not arguing that health insurance isn't helpful, or that it shouldn't be part of the solution. I'm saying that depending on our insurance-based healthcare model to address the chronic disease epidemic is misguided and shortsighted. The changes we need to make don't simply involve insuring more people, lowering the cost of prescription drugs, or mandating more twelve-minute "preventative check-ups." They are much more fundamental.

Today, we spend 86 percent of our healthcare dollars on treating chronic disease but just three percent on public health measures (NCCDPHP 2016). This gross imbalance nearly guarantees that our focus will remain on the far right end of the disease spectrum I introduced earlier in the book. Instead of preventing disease before it occurs, we're forced to spend our time and resources trying to mitigate its effects after it's firmly entrenched.

Preventing chronic disease before it occurs should always be the primary goal. But it's unrealistic to expect that we'll always be successful in that effort, which is why we also need a method for reversing it once it has taken hold. Our current approach to managing disease with drugs is not the answer. Instead, Functional Medicine offers a methodology for addressing the root cause of chronic problems, so patients can get well—and stay well—without unnecessary drugs and surgery.

Finally, we need a completely new model for delivering care. A brief appointment every six months is completely inadequate when the patient has multiple chronic diseases, is on multiple treatments, and is presenting with a new symptom. We can achieve the goal of true *health*care by connecting patients with a team of people who can work effectively with them on diet, lifestyle, and behavior change.

From Resistance to Revolution

Sounds good, right? So why isn't everybody already practicing this way?

There's a famous saying, often attributed to Arthur Schopenhauer: "All truth passes through three stages: First, it is ridiculed. Second, it is violently opposed. Third, it is accepted as being self-evident." For a while, Functional Medicine was ignored. More recently, some large conventional organizations have issued statements about Functional Medicine, a sign that it's starting to get traction. Some skeptics, and some conventional practitioners, still don't take Functional Medicine seriously. For many caregivers, however, this new model of healthcare is the self-evident solution to the current broken conventional model.

The launch of Cleveland Clinic Center for Functional Medicine has served to open many people's eyes to the potential of this model. Cleveland Clinic, as many people know, is a prestigious medical institution. They're often on the forefront of the newest treatments, therapies, and diagnostic procedures. In many ways, they're more progressive than the typical conventional establishment. The same is true for Mayo Clinic; they have a model that makes progressive care possible, as they're not beholden to some of the influences that limit progress in a conventional setting.

The mission of Cleveland Clinic Center for Functional Medicine, in addition to providing care for patients, is to do research on Functional Medicine that helps it to gain broader acceptance in the medical world. They've already taken some steps toward doing that, and have had promising results. Dr. Mark Hyman, the clinic director, travels all over the world to educate people about Functional Medicine. He's gone to places like Dubai, which is trying to set itself up as a center for medical tourism. They have expressed great interest in adopting Functional Medicine as the primary care model for delivering care to patients from all over the world, people who want to get the highest quality care and travel to Dubai for that reason.

Obviously, there's also a tremendous amount of interest in Functional Medicine from patients directly. Search volume for "Functional Medicine" on Google has nearly tripled in the past five years.

Google Trends

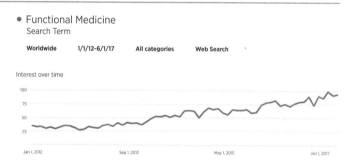

Search volume for "Functional Medicine" from 2012–2017

Well over a million people visit ChrisKresser.com and KresserInstitute.com each month, and we have nearly half a million email subscribers. Close to 400 practitioners have either already been trained or are in some stage of the ADAPT Practitioner Training Program at Kresser

Institute, with hundreds more training each month through the ADAPT Academy. Institute for Functional Medicine, the oldest international training organization for Functional Medicine, has trained thousands of practitioners from around the world.

Admittedly, Functional Medicine is still a niche. The average person on the street hasn't heard of it, but that's changing quickly. I've seen a difference even in the last three years. It doesn't take much for people to get excited about the concept once they're informed. When I explain Functional Medicine, they seem to immediately get it—it makes sense. Especially when we think of medical care in terms of analogies like the rock and the shoe, and the leaky boat, it's apparent which medical approach makes the most logical sense for patient health.

Doctors are often quick to buy in as well, even though they've typically been steeped in a conventional paradigm based in symptom suppression and disease management, rather than root cause resolution. Perhaps they are already feeling frustrated with a system that keeps them from making the impact they want to have on their patients. Some might be skeptical initially, but when they get some information on Functional Medicine, many doctors will ask for even more.

For these reasons, I firmly believe that the model we've

discussed in this book will eventually become the *de facto* way that medicine is practiced, both in this country and abroad. We won't refer to it as the ADAPT Framework or Functional Medicine because it will simply be woven into the fabric of the healthcare system. This transition won't happen overnight, and we'll face many significant challenges on the way. But we have no choice. The dramatic rise in chronic disease, coupled with the inadequacy of our current system to address it, demands that we adopt a new model, no matter how painful or difficult that might be initially. We owe it to ourselves, but perhaps most importantly, we owe it to our children and future generations.

On the Cutting Edge

Although the model discussed in this book hasn't yet become mainstream, there are several exciting examples of how it is being applied in today's healthcare landscape. Let's examine three case studies, each illustrating implementation of this approach in a different setting: a large institution, a primary care group, and a private clinic.

Cleveland Clinic

Cleveland Clinic's Center for Functional Medicine was spearheaded by Dr. Toby Cosgrove, the former president and CEO of Cleveland Clinic, and Dr. Mark Hyman, the chairman of Institute for Functional Medicine. Both are pioneers in the healthcare field. Dr. Cosgrove has been described as the "Wayne Gretsky of healthcare" (because he goes where the puck is going to be, not where it currently is). In other words, he's known for his ability to predict future trends and be on the forefront of those trends. Dr. Hyman, whom we met earlier in the book, has perhaps done more than any other person to advance and popularize Functional Medicine.

Cleveland Clinic has bet heavily on the success of Functional Medicine, investing tens of millions of dollars in their new center. They started out in a relatively small space with a few doctors but quickly outgrew it. Within months, they moved into a 17,000-square-foot facility in the renowned Glickman Tower, which houses the Cleveland Clinic cardiovascular and urology departments—both ranked number one in the world. They now have sixteen clinicians and over fifty employees and are continuing to grow at a breakneck pace.

That's a good thing because the demand from patients has been off the charts. At the time of this writing, they have a wait list of 2,600 patients from nine countries. Twenty-three percent of these patients are entirely new to Cleveland Clinic, which indicates that this new Center for Functional Medicine is driving demand.

They're also working in a cross-disciplinary way with other departments at Cleveland Clinic, exploring new models of care that group patients with doctors, nurse practitioners, nutritionists, and health coaches (similar to the collaborative model I've described in this book), performing research on the efficacy of Functional Medicine interventions and how they can reduce the cost of care, and even integrating nutrition and Functional Medicine curricula into the Cleveland Clinic Lerner College of Medicine.

The success of Cleveland Clinic's Center for Functional Medicine is perhaps the most exciting proof of concept we've seen yet because it demonstrates a strong demand for this type of medicine among patients, a recognition of its value by some of the most progressive thinkers in medicine, and the success of the model when implemented on a significant scale.

Iora Health

The second example is quite different from Cleveland Clinic but no less exciting. Iora Health is a primary care organization based in Denver, CO, and operating primarily in the Rocky Mountain region. They are blazing a trail in the collaborative care model; specifically, integrating health coaches into primary care.

Their focus is reversing type 2 diabetes with diet and lifestyle change. They achieve this not with lab testing and medications (though these are sometimes part of the treatment), but by teaming patients up with health coaches. Here's how it works.

They start by hiring coaches directly from the communities they will serve. This is important because it increases the likelihood that the coaches will be able to relate well to their clients and understand the challenges and obstacles that are specific to those communities. They don't hire people with significant experience or education in nutrition or healthcare. Instead, they screen for people who can form warm, empathetic connections with others. They've realized that this is the single most important quality that determines the success of a coaching intervention, and it's easier to train people in nutrition and lifestyle principles than it is to impart these relationship skills.

Once the coaches are trained, they begin working intensively with their clients. They teach them how to eat, go shopping with them, do pantry cleanouts, and even help them learn to cook and prepare foods with their new diet. They support them in adopting a new physical activity and exercise routine. They provide moral support and hold their client's hands through the entire process.

Another factor that sets Iora apart is their payment model. They accept "risk-adjusted, capitated fees," which is healthcare-speak for saying their compensation is performance-based: if they don't achieve the targets they set out, they don't receive full payment. On the other hand, if they exceed their targets, they earn a bonus. This performance-based pay structure, which is rare in mainstream medicine, has been adopted by many other progressive medical institutions as a way of controlling costs and improving the quality of care.

The Iora model has been incredibly successful. They're taking people from type 2 diabetes back to the pre-diabetic and even non-diabetic stage, and pre-diabetics back to non-diabetic blood sugar levels. What's more, they're doing this with minimal intervention from the physician. Patients do meet with the doctor for lab testing and a review of medications (if they're taking them), but these appointments are less frequent than they would be in a conventional model without health coaches. The primary relationship is between the patient and the coach, not the patient and the doctor—which, as I've argued throughout the book, is likely the best approach in cases where diet, behavior, and lifestyle change are the most important interventions.

Perhaps the best sign of Iora's success is how enthusiastic their patients are. The Net Promoter Score (NPS) is an index ranging from -100 to 100 that measures the willingness of customers to recommend a company's products or services to others. The national average NPS in primary care is four. The highest NPS in the traditional healthcare world is Kaiser Permanente, at 35. Apple, with its raving fans, has a NPS of 72. Iora's NPS is an impressive 90. They also boast a patient engagement score of 80 percent, versus the industry average of just 2 percent. These measurements show that Iora's patients are deeply engaged, satisfied, and highly likely to recommend the company to others.

Investors have also taken notice of Iora's success: Iora has raised over $30 million in venture capital, and venture capitalists are also investing in other similar models in this space.

California Center for Functional Medicine

My own clinic, California Center for Functional Medicine (CCFM), is an example of how the ADAPT Framework can be applied in the setting of a private, outpatient clinic. I was a solo practitioner using a "micropractice" approach for the first several years of my career. Initially, it was just myself and an office manager who doubled as a bookkeeper. After a couple years, I added a patient coordinator to provide more support to my patients, but I was still operating as a micropractice.

In 2014, I decided to join forces with Dr. Sunjya Schweig to create the California Center for Functional Medicine. Dr. Schweig and I shared a vision for creating a clinic that could support patients on a much larger scale, a place where we could implement many of the practices and principles that we've discussed throughout this book.

Just three years later, CCFM now has four clinicians, a nurse practitioner, a health coach, two nutritionists, an administrative staff of thirteen, and thousands of patients. We've developed a care model that incorporates the three elements of the ADAPT Framework: Functional Medicine, an ancestral diet and lifestyle, and a collaborative practice structure.

Patients start their work with us via a thirty-minute telephone or videoconference appointment, which we call the Initial Consult. The Initial Consult is conducted by a nurse practitioner, who collects the patient's chief complaints or primary goals for working with us, documents relevant background and history, orders the necessary laboratory tests, and sends the detailed new patient intake paperwork. The nurse practitioner will also make diet and lifestyle recommendations for the patient to start with while she is completing the labs and waiting for her first in-person appointment. This means that the patient can make meaningful progress before she has even seen the clinician, either on her own or under the guidance of the nurse practitioner and the health coach.

Once the tests have been completed and the results are in—usually about six to eight weeks after the Initial Consult—the patient has their Case Review. This is an in-person, sixty to seventy-five-minute appointment in our office. Prior to the appointment, the clinician will have reviewed the patient's intake paperwork (electronically, of course) and lab test results, and prepared a "report of findings" that summarizes the underlying patterns contributing to the patient's complaints, recommendations for further testing if necessary, and outlining the treatment plan. The clinician then presents this report of findings to the patient, answers any questions they have, and explains how the treatment process will work.

Patients love the Case Review. We consistently hear comments like, "No one has ever taken the time to put these pieces together," and, "I finally feel like someone is seeing the full picture," and, "I feel hopeful for the first time in years because I now understand the causes of my symptoms and what to do about them." The clinicians at CCFM also love the Case Review process because it provides us the time and information we need to make more accurate diagnoses and create more effective treatment plans. It also offers plenty of time for us to interact with the patient, answer questions, and build a relationship that will support long-term health and well-being.

At the end of the Case Review, the clinician will suggest that the patient schedule a check-in with the nurse practitioner every two weeks, for as long as the patient is on a protocol. These check-ins provide a means for addressing any side effects or difficulties the patient may be having with the protocol and answering any questions that the patient may have. The clinician may also refer the patient to our health coach, who can provide a deeper level of assistance with the diet, lifestyle, and behavior changes the clinician recommended. Our patients tend to be highly motivated, especially compared to the general population, so not all of them need or want this support. But it's extremely helpful for those who do.

We also offer standalone appointments with the health coach, and with our two staff nutritionists. These can be helpful for our patients who are no longer on an intensive protocol but are still addressing lingering symptoms or optimizing their health and need additional support.

In addition to the live, human support mentioned above,

we've developed over a hundred patient handouts on topics ranging from the Low FODMAP diet, to FAQs on how to properly prepare for and perform the lab tests that we prescribe, to strategies for stress management. These handouts support patient compliance and can also reduce the number of questions that the clinicians and administrative staff would otherwise receive, thus lowering overhead.

We've also started developing six- to eight-week classes/ groups on specific health topics, such as weight loss, autoimmune disease, pain relief, and fertility. These classes, which will be offered both locally and virtually, are efficient ways of delivering additional education and tools to patients with similar needs. They're also a way of building community and reducing the isolation and loneliness that often accompanies chronic disease.

At the time of this writing, we're developing a wellness program for the local fire department in Berkeley, CA. They reached out for help with their newest recruits. Their goals were to learn skills and techniques for better performance, reduce workers' compensation injuries, reduce the amount of sick days, increase mental and physical wellbeing, and to provide long-term tools for sustainability to take with them throughout their career. We created a program that includes a whole foods, nutrient-dense diet, bodyweight training exercises, stress management and meditation, and improved sleep hygiene. We'll be incorporating blood tests, continuous glucose monitors, and other hardware devices that monitor steps, sleep patterns, and heart rate variability to track their progress.

These examples suggest that the ADAPT Framework principles we've discussed throughout the book are applicable in a wide variety of settings, ranging from large institutions like Cleveland Clinic, to regional primary care groups like Iora Health, to private outpatient clinics like California Center for Functional Medicine. This is truly the future of medicine!

CHAPTER SIXTEEN

NEXT STEPS: THREE THINGS TO DO NOW

First, thank you for reading this book. I know that your time is precious, and I know how many other books are out there. Thank you for choosing this one.

Whether you're a healthcare practitioner, a student, someone trying to address a chronic health problem, or a "citizen scientist" and health enthusiast, I hope this book has inspired you to get involved. I've listed three steps below that you can take right now, regardless of your background, to start your journey.

1) Download a Free Bonus Chapter

I've done my best to paint a clear picture in this book of what the ADAPT Framework looks like in practice. But the best way to see it in action is with detailed case studies of real patients I've worked with in my clinic, including their symptoms and complaints, the lab tests I ordered, the results of those tests and how I interpreted those results, my diagnosis, the treatment protocols I prescribed, and the results of the treatment. These case studies would have made the book about 30 percent longer, and a lot of the lab results wouldn't display well in a book format. So, I've decided to make them available (exclusively to readers of this book) as a free bonus chapter.

You can download it at **UnconventionalMedicineBook. com/bonus.**

2) Get Personalized Recommendations

If you're ready to take the next step, your path forward will depend upon whether you're a practitioner or layperson, and your needs and goals. For example, if you're a medical doctor currently practicing within a primary care setting, and this book was your first exposure to Functional Medicine and ancestral diet and lifestyle, my suggestions for you will be different than if you're a health coach who is already quite familiar with these concepts. Likewise, if you're not a practitioner, my recommendations will vary based on whether you're trying to address a chronic disease, optimize your health, or just help spread the message in this book and reinvent healthcare.

To that end, I've created a free online assessment to provide you with recommendations that are customized for your specific situation.

To take the assessment, visit UnconventionalMedicineBook.com/assessment.

3) Get Educated and Learn More

If you're new to this approach, one of the best ways to determine whether it's right for you is to take a deeper dive into each of the elements of the ADAPT Framework we've discussed in the book: Functional Medicine, ancestral health, and a collaborative practice model.

In the next chapter, I've outlined some of my favorite websites, books, podcasts, and training resources in these areas. It's not an exhaustive list, but it's enough to give you a big head start on your journey.

A Note About Going Against the Grain

Functional Medicine and the ancestral diet and lifestyle have exploded in popularity over the past several years, and current trends suggest that interest in these areas will only continue to grow.

That said, although the ideas we've discussed throughout the book are well supported by both evidence and common sense, they're still firmly outside of the dominant medical paradigm. If you do choose to pursue this path, know that you are likely to meet resistance and skepticism—from colleagues or supervisors at work, and perhaps even friends or family members.

Remember Arthur Schopenhauer's famous saying about the stages that a new idea must pass through before it is accepted? If we understand the truth of this, we can be more prepared to meet the resistance and skepticism when they inevitably come. We can see them for what they are and take them in stride, rather than letting them derail us from our path.

For example, I was recently uninvited—after being initially accepted as a speaker—to a national health conference. I was planning to give a talk that covered many of the concepts I've presented in this book. Although I wasn't directly given a specific reason why I was uninvited, I heard through the grapevine that it was because certain conservative members of the organization putting on the conference were not supportive of some of the ideas in my talk.

Fortunately, although we can expect to meet this kind of resistance as we blaze a new trail, we can also expect our ideas to be received with enthusiasm and a recognition of their importance and worth. This, in fact, is the most common response I encounter when I speak about the ADAPT Framework at conferences, to doctors and other healthcare providers, and to the public. Most doctors know from their own experience that we're failing to address chronic disease and provide patients with the solutions they seek. This is even more self-evident to patients, since they're the ones struggling each day with the very real consequences of this failure.

And while those of us who have embraced this vision of reinventing healthcare and ending chronic disease may still be in the minority, we can take heart in the immortal words of Margaret Mead:

> "Never doubt that a small group of thoughtful, committed citizens can change the world. Indeed, it is the only thing that ever has."

CHAPTER SEVENTEEN

RESOURCES FOR PRACTITIONERS & PATIENTS

There are many entry paths for practitioners interested in Functional Medicine and an ancestral diet and lifestyle in general, or the ADAPT Framework specifically.

Kresser Institute

The ADAPT Framework informs the programs at Kresser Institute, and we offer several options.

ADAPT Academy

ADAPT Academy was created specifically for people who are interested in the ADAPT Framework approach but are not yet sure they want to do a full training program or spend several thousand dollars traveling to a conference. For those who can't immediately commit significant time, money, and professional investment, the Academy enables people to "dip their toes" into the approach. It offers the opportunity to start some training and begin meeting people who are already involved in this framework. It puts medical professionals in contact with others who share their interests and enables participants to acquire some skills, practical tools, and resources that can be put into practice right away with patients.

ADAPT Academy is offered through a monthly online membership platform. It features:

- **Live seminars** with guest experts on specific topics, such as "Treating Very High LDL-P" with Dr. Tom Dayspring, "Updated SIBO Guidelines" with Dr. Mark Pimentel, and "Evidence-Based Strategies for Assessing the HPA Axis" with Mark Newman. Participants can interact with the expert and ask questions, and handouts, cheat sheets, and other tools to help with implementation are provided.

- **4–12-week, in-depth courses** covering key areas of interest for practitioners. Examples include In Practice, a series on treating the ten most common conditions we see in practice from a Functional Medicine perspective; a seminar on diagnosing and treating SIBO; and Busy to Balanced, a course on mastering productivity and time management.

- **Quick Wins**, which are short lessons that contain immediately applicable information and tools that you can start using in your practice right away. For example, we might talk about a new lab test that's become available and how to interpret it and use it with your patients. I might tell you about an excellent form of glutathione supplement to use in your practice, how to use it, and why. We might discuss a new piece of software that's become available to improve practice management and administration. The Quick Wins are all viewable in five to ten minutes and are highly focused on practical application.

- **Research Updates** with the latest research grouped according to specific topics, e.g., "Autoimmune Disease," "Metabolic Syndrome," and "Environmental Toxins." These not only provide summaries of the most recent research but more importantly an analysis of how the research is relevant to clinical practice. Instead of just citing a study, we distill the most important points and translate them into practical steps that can be immediately applied in a clinical setting.

- **An active forum** with people from all over the world who are starting to incorporate the ADAPT Framework into their practice. Networking sessions link up coaches and other allied providers who are hoping to work with licensed clinicians, and vice versa.

The Academy is not just for licensed clinicians but is also a hub for other providers, such as nurse practitioners and physician assistants, along with anyone considering a career in this field. Medical students, or students in a chiropractic or acupuncture program, for example, may benefit from the opportunities available through the Academy. Practicing health coaches and people currently working toward their health coaching or nutrition certification would likewise be welcome and encouraged to participate at the Academy.

ADAPT Practitioner Training Program

We also offer the ADAPT Practitioner Training Program, which is designed to provide practitioners with everything they need to start a successful Functional Medicine practice, incorporating an ancestral diet and lifestyle and a collaborative practice model. Not surprisingly, the program has three tracks. One track is Functional Medicine, which is broken into three key areas: Gut, HPA Axis, and Blood Chemistry. The second track concentrates on the Exposome: an ancestral diet and lifestyle. The third track covers practice management, the specific knowledge and tools required to set up and run a successful Functional Medicine practice—information that is very different from running a conventional medicine practice.

The ADAPT Practitioner Training Program requires a more significant commitment than the Academy. It's a twelve-month program, which requires three to six hours a week of participation. It's been highly successful with almost 400 clinicians from around the world who have either completed the training or are currently enrolled.

ADAPT Health Coach Training Program

In the spring of 2018, we'll launch the ADAPT Health Coach Training Program, which will train health coaches in our ADAPT model. We'll teach them how to work with clients on the ancestral diet and lifestyle. We won't be covering how to interpret labs or how to prescribe treatment—areas that are the province of licensed pro-viders—but we'll be teaching them the basic principles of Functional Medicine. We'll also be educating them to support clients in making behavior changes. They'll learn the fascinating research on the evidence-based principles of behavior change and will be trained in effectively supporting people using a coaching model, rather than relying exclusively on the expert model.

In other words, instead of telling patients what to do and expecting that they're going to do it, this coaching model uses the principles of coaching psychology and behavior change to help patients be successful. There will also be professional development training for coaches with information on how to work with licensed providers like doctors and other medical professionals; how to get a job within a Functional Medicine clinic; what it's like working there once you're in; and how to start your own practice.

The Health Coach Training Program will be offered in two tracks: certification, for those who want the highest level of training and recognition, and non-certification, for those who wish to learn the material but are not interested in or ready for certification.

Live Events and Advanced Modules

In addition to the programs just mentioned, in 2018, Kresser Institute will begin offering live, in-person events and advanced modules on specific topics. The live events will give practitioners, coaches, and other people training within the Kresser Institute and ADAPT Framework ecosystem a chance to meet in person, network, collaborate, and gain additional skills and tools that benefit from a physical presence.

The advanced modules will cover topics not taught in the core Practitioner and Health Coach Training Programs but that are of interest to practitioners and coaches working within the ADAPT Framework. Examples might include modules on chronic infection, detoxification, and hormones for practitioners, and modules on developing group programs and using genetic information to customize diet and lifestyle recommendations for coaches.

You can learn more about ADAPT Academy, the Practitioner and Health Coach Training, and other Kresser Institute programs at KresserInstitute.com.

Other Training
Institute for Functional Medicine (IFM)

IFM has been training practitioners in Functional Medicine for twenty-five years. They offer seminars in person in the U.S. and U.K., and via livestream format. Topics include cardiovascular health, digestive health, genetics, immune/autoimmune, detoxification, and applying functional medicine in clinical practice. Seminars can be taken on a modular basis, and IFM also offers a certification track for practitioners who want to go deeper with the training.

You can learn more about IFM training at Functional-Medicine.org.

Kalish Institute

Kalish Institute was created by Dan Kalish, DC, a chiropractor who has been practicing and teaching Functional Medicine for more than twenty years. Kalish Institute training is offered online and includes programs on Functional Medicine basics, practice management, gut health, and hormones, as well as a six-month "virtual mentorship." Like Kresser Institute programs, Kalish Institute offerings emphasize case studies and practical application, which is particularly helpful for practitioners new to Functional Medicine.

You can learn more about Kalish Institute training at KalishInstitute.com.

Masterclass with Masterjohn Pro

These series of "masterclasses" with Dr. Chris Masterjohn, a nutritional scientist, go into great depth on topics like energy metabolism—topics we all learned while studying medicine but may need a refresher on. Chris hits the science hard, but he also takes the time to explain why it's relevant and how you can apply it in clinical practice. The classes are available online and include video, audio, slides, and transcripts in PDF format.

You can learn more about Masterclass with Masterjohn Pro at ChrisMasterjohnPhD.com/pro.

Websites, Podcasts, and Books

In addition to the more in-depth educational opportunities listed above, there are many websites, podcasts and books that cover topics related to Functional Medicine and an ancestral diet and lifestyle.

Websites

KresserInstitute.com

This is the website and blog for Kresser Institute. The blog features regular articles pertaining to all three elements of the ADAPT Framework: Functional Medicine, an ancestral diet and lifestyle, and collaborative practice model.

KresserInstitute.com is geared specifically toward healthcare practitioners. Recent articles include "Does Testosterone Therapy Increase the Risk of Heart Disease in Men?,"

"Treating Methylation: Are We Over-supplementing?," and "Research Studies: Why the Media So Often Gets Them Wrong." The articles at KresserInstitute.com typically provide additional information of interest to providers on disease processes, mechanisms, and treatment.

ChrisKresser.com

My primary website and blog. Although not specifically geared toward practitioners, much of the content is directly relevant to that audience. Blog articles cover the ancestral diet and lifestyle, the latest research in medicine and health, Functional Medicine approaches to common conditions, and more. ChrisKresser.com also offers a variety of free eBooks and special reports on specific topics, such as gut health, thyroid disorders, and weight loss. Recent articles include "How Many Steps Should You Get in a Day?," "Resolving the Underlying Causes of ADHD," and "Could Type 1 Diabetes Be Reversible After All?"

14Four.me

If you or your patients need help implementing the ancestral diet and lifestyle I've mentioned in this book but don't have access to a health coach trained in these areas, check out 14Four. The purpose of the program is to help people make effective change in four key areas:

diet, sleep, physical activity, and stress management. We help the patient reboot their diet. We help them to move more like their ancestors. We help them to manage their stress, and they get more restorative sleep. The website offers videos, audio programs, and handouts to make implementation easier. The program itself is two weeks, but it's preceded by a two-week "on ramp" and followed by a one-week wind-down, so it takes five weeks to complete. Thousands of people around the world have used 14Four to dramatically improve their overall health and even reverse chronic diseases.

Examine.com

Examine.com was created by a group of scientists and researchers with the mission of delivering independent and critical analysis of current research in the fields of nutrition and medicine—a service that has been sorely lacking until now. Mainstream media reporting on recent research is often incomplete or even misleading; it seems that there are few true science journalists left who can critically examine a study, evaluate its claims, and report on it in a comprehensive yet accessible way. Examine. com does this incredibly well. You can read their blog for free, or sign up for their subscription service, which provides in-depth coverage of the most recent research for a reasonable fee.

StephanGuyenet.com

Dr. Stephan Guyenet is a scientist who formerly studied the neurobiology of weight regulation at the University of Washington. He has also written a blog for many years, summarizing and analyzing the most recent research on a wide variety of topics related to obesity, diabetes, metabolism, nutrition, and optimal health. Stephan is one of the most lucid and balanced voices in the field, and his book *The Hungry Brain: Outsmarting the Instincts That Make Us Overeat* is a must-read for anyone wishing to truly understand the science behind fat loss and weight regulation.

ChrisMasterjohnPhD.com

I mentioned Dr. Chris Masterjohn earlier. He's a nutritional scientist who has recently left academia to pursue his own research and develop educational programs for consumers and professionals. Chris is one of the brightest minds I've ever encountered in this space, and he is widely known for his deep dives into the science and his ability to translate that understanding into practical and actionable advice for both clinicians and patients. He has a blog and podcast, which can be found at his website.

RobbWolf.com

If you've been following the Paleo and ancestral health

movement for any length of time, you've no doubt heard of Robb Wolf. A former research biochemist, Robb has perhaps done more than anyone to increase awareness of the importance of an ancestral perspective for both health optimization and disease prevention and reversal. Robb is known for his no-nonsense approach and his encyclopedic knowledge of a wide range of topics, including diet and nutrition, physical activity, sustainability and food systems, and nutritional science. He has a blog, wildly popular podcast, and two books, all of which can be found at his website.

MarksDailyApple.com

Mark's Daily Apple was created by Mark Sisson, a former competitive triathlete and fitness expert. He writes and speaks about what he calls the "Primal" diet and lifestyle, which is his term for the ancestral approach we've discussed in this book. Mark is known for his accessible and level-headed style, and his blog is one of the most popular and highly accessed natural health websites in the world. Mark also founded a company called Primal Nutrition, which has a fantastic line of food products such as salad dressings, mayo, and bars made with "Primal-friendly" ingredients. You can find Mark's blog, several books, podcast, and food products at his website.

DrHyman.com

Together with Dr. Jeffrey Bland, who founded IFM in the 1990s, Dr. Mark Hyman has been a prolific ambassador of Functional Medicine and has arguably done more than anyone else to advance it. Dr. Hyman, a physician, is the director of Cleveland Clinic Center for Functional Medicine, which we discussed earlier in this book. He's also the author of ten #1 *New York Times* best-selling books on nutrition and health, and has a popular blog, podcast, YouTube channel, and social media presence.

SaraGottfried.com

Dr. Sara Gottfried, a Harvard-trained MD, has turned her focus to educating the public on health and wellness, with a focus on women's health and using genetics and epigenetics to improve well-being and extend lifespan. Sara is known for both her rigorous approach to the science and her warm, accessible style—a rare combination that has earned her hundreds of thousands of loyal fans around the world. She has a blog, several books, and programs available at her website.

Conferences

In addition to the websites, books, and podcasts mentioned above, there are several conferences that cover Functional Medicine and the ancestral diet and lifestyle.

Kresser Institute

In 2018, Kresser Institute will hold its first annual conference, featuring presentations, workshops, and experiential
breakout groups on a wide range of topics within the
ADAPT Framework: Functional Medicine, ancestral
health, and the collaborative practice model. Consistent with the mission of Kresser Institute, the training at
the conference will be highly practical and "hands on,"
with an emphasis on applying what is learned in a clinical
setting. Networking sessions with licensed clinicians and
allied providers, health coaches, and nutritionists will
be offered, to facilitate the collaborative practice model
endorsed by the ADAPT Framework.

Find out more at KresserInstitute.com

Ancestral Health Symposium

The Ancestral Health Symposium (AHS) is the premier
academic conference covering topics related to the ancestral diet and lifestyle principles discussed in this book. It
is typically held in August or September at a university
in the U.S. and draws well-known speakers in the field
from all over the world. The presentations are oriented
toward scientists, clinicians, practitioners, and "citizen scientists," members of the public who follow these
topics closely.

Find out more AncestralHealth.org.

Paleo f(x)

Where AHS has a more academic focus, Paleo f(x) has always emphasized translating theory into practice. Since it started in 2013, it has quickly become the most popular and widely attended conference in this space. Spanning over three days (held in Austin, TX), Paleo f(x) features multiple stages and a massive vendor fair. It has an array of keynote presentations, mastermind panels, cooking demos, and workshops, all led by cutting-edge health practitioners, scientists in a variety of fields, coaches and gym owners, *New York Times* best-selling authors, popular bloggers, community and sustainability activists, biohackers, chefs, and more.

Visit Paleofx.com for more info.

IFM Annual Conference

IFM holds its Annual International Conference (AIC) in June each year. The AIC features presentations and other learning sessions by some of the top speakers in the field, typically organized around a theme. For example, in 2017, the theme was how neuroplasticity can be harnessed and optimized to prevent and treat neurodegenerative diseases, brain injury, stroke, and mental disorders. The IFM AIC is a great opportunity to meet and network with other clinicians and allied providers from around the world who have embraced a Functional Medicine approach.

Visit IFM.org/ifm-planning-calendar for more info.

Podcasts

Revolution Health Radio

This is my podcast. I cover a wide range of topics related to Functional Medicine and a genetically-aligned diet and lifestyle, interview guest experts, and answer listener questions. Episodes are between twenty minutes and one hour, and the show is available on iTunes (where it is consistently in the Top 5 of all podcasts in the Alternative Health category) and on my website.

You can download the podcasts and read transcripts at ChrisKresser.com/category/podcasts.

Other podcasts

Many of the experts I mentioned above also have podcasts, including Mark Sisson, Robb Wolf, and Chris Masterjohn. You can find them at their websites, or on iTunes.

Books

There are far too many good books to list here, so I've included a small but representative sample of titles that cover the ancestral diet and lifestyle in more depth and illustrate the Functional Medicine approach to chronic disease.

The Paleo Cure

My first book, *The Paleo Cure* (published in hardcover as *Your Personal Paleo Code*), uses the Paleo diet as a template from which you can tailor a simple yet powerful three-step program—Reset, Rebuild, Revive—to fit your lifestyle, body type, and genetic blueprint. It shows you how to eliminate the toxic foods that cause illness and weight gain, how to sleep better, exercise like our ancestors, cultivate pleasure, and vastly improve overall health. It also teaches you how to personalize your prescription by addressing specific health conditions, from heart disease to digestive problems. You can find *The Paleo Cure* at bookstores, on Amazon, and at PaleoCureBook.com.

The End of Alzheimer's: The First Program to Prevent and Reverse Cognitive Decline

This seminal book by Alzheimer's researcher and physician Dr. Dale Bredesen will forever change the way we look at this horrific disease. Dr. Bredesen describes a Functional Medicine approach to preventing and treating Alzheimer's disease, offering hope for the first time to the millions of people around the world who've been diagnosed with this condition and told there is nothing they can do. His book is available in bookstores and on Amazon.

The Wahls Protocol: A Radical New Way to Treat All Chronic Autoimmune Conditions Using Paleo Principles

Dr. Wahls reversed her progressive MS—going from being wheelchair-bound to completing an eighteen-mile bicycle tour—in less than twelve months using principles of Functional Medicine and an ancestral diet and lifestyle. Her book is an inspiring and helpful guide for anyone who is suffering from autoimmune disease and looking for an alternative to conventional, symptom-based treatment.

Brain Maker: The Power of Gut Microbes to Heal and Protect Your Brain—for Life

This book, by board-certified neurologist and four-time *New York Times* best-selling author Dr. David Perlmutter, explains the potent interplay between intestinal microbes and the brain, describing how the microbiome develops from birth and evolves based on lifestyle choices, how it can become "sick," and how nurturing gut health through a few easy strategies can alter your brain's destiny for the better. It's another fantastic example of how a Functional Medicine approach can be applied to conditions that are poorly treated by conventional medicine.

Resources for Patients

What about patients who want to pursue healing in a Functional Medicine setting? If you're struggling with a chronic health challenge, and you want to find a clinician to work with, there are a few different options to pursue.

Finding a Functional Medicine practitioner

First, at the Kresser Institute website, we have a practitioner directory listing practitioners who have been trained in the ADAPT Framework.

You can find it at KresserInstitute.com/directory.

Second, IFM also has a practitioner directory, noting those who have done some of their trainings, along with people who have gone through their entire certification process. IFM doesn't necessarily embrace the ancestral perspective or the collaborative practice model, so IFM-trained practitioners might offer a slightly different approach than what's been outlined in this book. That said, IFM has trained several excellent, qualified practitioners, and is therefore a good source for people who are looking for someone trained in Functional Medicine. Lest we forget, there's also Google. Simply performing a Google search for a Functional Medicine doctor or physician in your town is another option.

Patients play a vital role in leading this revolution toward Functional Medicine and the ancestral diet and lifestyle. The only way some doctors hear about it is from their patients. I hear this from Kresser Institute training program participants all the time. Some patients may feel hesitant to talk to their doctors about it. If a patient already has a good relationship with his or her doctor, and the doctor is open-minded and willing to hear about other approaches, then bringing it up can help pave the way toward a new model of healthcare.

Finding a Health Coach

Working with a health coach is another great option. Kresser Institute will eventually offer a low-cost clinic with sessions with students in the Kresser Institute Health Coach Training Program.

The coaches coming out of Kresser Institute will have

awareness of this evolutionary perspective, which is a key criterion to look for in a health coach. Any health coach who just provides information isn't doing enough. Patients should also look for coaches with training in psychology and behavior change. Ideally, a coach should work collaboratively with their patients; this requires a thorough understanding of how to facilitate behavior change, and training in disciplines like positive psychology, strengths-based coaching, and motivational interviewing.

Patients can find a health coach through several resources. As mentioned above, in 2018 Kresser Institute will be launching the ADAPT Health Coach Training Program. Once the first group of ADAPT Health Coaches is certified, they will be listed in a directory at KresserInstitute.com.

In the meantime, you can search for coaches by contacting coaching programs that have been approved by prominent accreditation organizations. The best known of these for health coaching programs is the International Consortium for Health and Wellness Coaching. They have robust requirements and a board exam that qualified coaches can sit for to become certified. There is also the International Coaching Federation, which has a directory of people who have been certified through them. Health coaches who possess certification from either institution will likely be trustworthy in their skill and knowledge.

As the Functional Medicine model moves more and more into the mainstream, we have an opportunity to stem the tide of chronic diseases that are shortening our lifespans and destroying our quality of life. I believe that the approach I've outlined in this book is the best chance we have to address the problem of chronic illness, both on an individual level and on a societal level. We need to do that for our own benefit and for the benefit of our children.

ACKNOWLEDGMENTS

I've heard it said that it takes a village to write a book. That's certainly true in this case. To my beloved wife, Elanne, thank you for your wisdom, support, and flexibility as I wrangled with this project (and several others at the same time). I couldn't have done it without you. To my precious daughter, Sylvie, thanks for putting up with the changes in our normal routine—I missed some of our sweet mornings together as the deadline approached. Thank you, Jon and Keith, for your guidance and feedback, especially at the eleventh hour.

I'd like to thank my friend and colleague Dr. Mark Hyman, for writing the foreword, and being a trailblazer and source of inspiration in this field. A big shout out to my editorial team—Hal, Sheila, and Jeremy—for their contribution and professionalism. Thank you to the clinicians who generously shared their stories for the book.

To my co-workers and colleagues at CKLLC and CCFM, thank you for your hard work and dedication to our purpose of ending chronic disease. Thank you to the practitioners training at Kresser Institute for joining the fight and putting your faith in the ADAPT Framework, and in me. Finally, a deep and humble thank you to my many patients over the years for your trust in me and for being my greatest teachers. I wouldn't be here without you.

REFERENCES

Alzheimer's Association. 2017. *2017 Alzheimer's Disease Facts and Figures*. Accessed August 17, 2017. http://www.alz.org/facts/.

American Autoimmune Related Disease Association (AARDA). 2017. *Autoimmune Statistics*. August. Accessed August 17, 2017. https://www.aarda.org/news-information/statistics/#14882343 45559-44c8ff57-216d.

American College of Preventive Medicine (ACPM). 2009. *Lifestyle Medicine—Evidence Review*. Accessed July 21, 2017. https:// health.uconn.edu/student-wellness/wp-content/uploads/ sites/170/2017/08/WellnessSitePage102Attachment1.pdf.

Appel, Lawrence J., et al. 2011. "Comparative Effectiveness of Weight-Loss Interventions in Clinical Practice." *The New England Journal of Medicine* 365: 1959–1968. Accessed August 17, 2017. http://www.nejm.org/doi/full/10.1056/ NEJMoa1108660#t=articl.

Asgary, S., et al. 2017. "Serum Levels of Lead, Mercury and Cadmium in Relation to Coronary Artery Disease in the Elderly: A Cross-Sectional Study." *Chemosphere* 180: 540–544. Accessed August 17, 2017. https://www.ncbi.nlm.nih.gov/pubmed/28431391.

Begley, C. Glenn, and Lee M. Ellis. 2012. "Drug Development: Raise Standards for Preclinical Cancer Research." *Nature* 483 (7391): 531–533. Accessed August 17, 2017. http://www.nature.com/nature/journal/v483/n7391/full/483531a.html?foxtrotcallback=true.

Bhatia, Aatish. 2012. "Milk, Meat and Blood: How Diet Drives Natural Selection in the Maasai." *Wired.com.* September 30. Accessed July 21, 2017. https://www.wired.com/2012/09/milk-meat-and-blood-how-diet-drives-natural-selection-in-the-maasai/.

Bird, J.K., et al. 2017. "Risk of Deficiency in Multiple Concurrent Micronutrients in Children and Adults in the United States." *Nutrients* 9 (7). Accessed August 17, 2017. https://www.ncbi.nlm.nih.gov/pubmed/28672791.

Blask, David E., et al. 2009. "Melatonin, Sleep Disturbance and Cancer Risk." *Sleep Medicine Reviews* 13 (4): 257–264. Accessed August 17, 2017. https://blog.lsgc.com/wp-content/uploads/2016/04/05.-Blask-Melatonin-Cancer-Review.pdf.

Bowe, Whitney P., and Alan C. Logan. 2011. "Acne Vulgaris, Pro- biotics and the Gut-Brain-Skin Axis: Back to the Future?" *Gut Pathogens* 3 (1). Accessed August 17, 2017. https://gutpathogens.biomedcentral.com/articles/10.1186/1757-4749-3-1.

Bredesen, Dale. 2017. *The End of Alzheimer's: The First Program to Prevent and Reverse Cognitive Decline.* New York: Avery.

Brody, Jane E. 2017. "Learning From Our Parents' Heart Health Mistakes." *The New York Times.* April 10, 2017. Accessed July 21, 2017. https://www.nytimes.com/2017/04/10/well/live/learning-from-our-parents-heart-health-mistakes.html.

Brown, Troy. 2015. "100 Best-Selling, Most Prescribed Branded Drugs Through March." *Medscape News & Perspective.* May 6, 2015. Accessed July 22, 2017. http://www.medscape.com/viewarticle/844317.

Butterworth, S., et al. 2006. "Effect of Motivational Interviewing-Based Health Coaching on Employees' Physical and Mental Health Status." *Journal of Occupational Health Psychology* 11 (4): 358–65. Accessed August 17, 2017. https://www.ncbi.nlm.nih.gov/pubmed/17059299.

Catassi, C., et al. 1995. "High Prevalence of Undiagnosed Coeliac Disease in 5280 Italian Students Screened by Antigliadin Antibodies." *Acta Paediatrica* 84 (6): 672–6. Accessed August 17, 2017. http://pmid.us/7670254.

Centers for Disease Control and Prevention (CDC). 2011. *Asthma in the US.* May 2011. Accessed August 17, 2017. https://www.cdc.gov/vitalsigns/asthma/index.html.

—. 2015. *Health, United States 2015: With Special Feature on Racial and Ethnic Health Disparities.* Accessed July 24, 2017. https://www.cdc.gov/nchs/data/hus/hus15.pdf.

—. 2016. "Infertility." *CDC National Center for Health Statistics.* Accessed July 24, 2017. https://www.cdc.gov/nchs/fastats/infertility.htm.

—. 2017a. *Attention Deficit/Hyperactivity Disorder (ADHD) Data & Statistics.* July 18. Accessed July 21, 2017. https://www.cdc.gov/ncbddd/adhd/data.html.

—. 2017b. *New CDC Report: More Than 100 Million Americans Have Diabetes or Prediabetes.* July 18. Accessed August 17, 2017. https://www.cdc.gov/media/releases/2017/p0718-diabetes-report.html.

Centers for Medicare & Medicaid Services (CMS). 2015. *Chronic Conditions.* Accessed August 17, 2017. https://www.cms.gov/Research-Statistics-Data-and-Systems/Statistics-Trends-and-Reports/Chronic-Conditions/CC_Main.html.

Chen, Pauline W. 2013. "For New Doctors, 8 Minutes Per Patient." *The New York Times.* May 30, 2013. Accessed August 17, 2017. https://well.blogs.nytimes.com/2013/05/30/for-new-doctors-8-minutes-per-patient/?_r=0.

Chepesiuk, R. 2009. "Missing the Dark: Health Effects of Light Pollution." *Environmental Health Perspectives* 117 (1): A20–27. Accessed August 17, 2017. https://www.ncbi.nlm.nih.gov/pmc/articles/PMC2627884/.

Choy, C.M., et al. 2002. "Infertility, Blood Mercury Concentrations and Dietary Seafood Consumption: A Case-Control Study." *BJOG: An International Journal of Obstetrics & Gynaecology* 109 (10): 1121–5. Accessed August 17, 2017. https://www.ncbi.nlm.nih.gov/pubmed/12387464.

Cordain, Loren, and Joe Friel. 2005. *The Paleo Diet for Athletes: A Nutritional Formula for Peak Athletic Performance*. New York: Rodale Books.

Cowen, Philip J., and Michael Browning. 2015. "What Has Serotonin to Do with Depression?" *World Psychiatry* 14 (2): 158–60. Accessed August 17, 2017. https://www.ncbi.nlm.nih.gov/pmc/articles/PMC4471964/.

Crimmins, Eileen M., et al. 2016. "Trends Over 4 Decades in Disability-Free Life Expectancy in the United States." *American Journal of Public Health* 106 (7): 1287–93. Accessed August 17, 2017. https://www.ncbi.nlm.nih.gov/pubmed/27077352.

Daniels, Judith K., et al. 2017. "Depressed Gut: The Microbiota-Diet-Inflammation Trialogue in Depression." *Current Opinion in Psychiatry* 30 (5): 369–377. Accessed July 24, 2017. http://journals.lww.com/co-psychiatry/Abstract/publishahead/Depressed_gut__The_microbiota_diet_inflammation.99348.aspx.

Dietary Guidelines Advisory Committee (DIAG). 2010. *Report of the Dietary Guidelines Advisory Committee. Nutriwatch.org.* Accessed July 21, 2017. https://www.nutriwatch.org/05Guidelines/dga_advisory_2010.pdf.

Duff-Brown, Beth. 2017. "Non-Communicable Disease Could Cost $47 Trillion by 2030." *Stanford FSI News.* March 7. Accessed August 2, 2017. http://fsi.stanford.edu/news/non-communical-disease-could-cost-47-trillion-2030.

Dukowicz, Andrew C., et al. 2007. "Small Intestinal Bacterial Over-growth." *Gastroenterology & Hepatology* 3 (2): 112–122. Accessed August 17, 2017. https://www.ncbi.nlm.nih.gov/pmc/articles/PMC3099351/.

Elfhaq, K., and S. Rossner. 2005. "Who Succeeds in Maintaining Weight Loss? A Conceptual Review of Factors Associated with Weight Loss Maintenance and Weight Regain." *Obesity Reviews* 6 (1): 67–85. Accessed August 17, 2017. https://www.ncbi.nlm.nih.gov/pubmed/15655039.

Fasano, A., and C. Catassi. 2001. "Current Approaches to Diagnosis and Treatment of Celiac Disease: An Evolving Spectrum." *Gastroenterology* 120 (3): 636–51. Accessed August 17, 2017. http://pmid.us/11179241.

Fournier, J.C., et al. 2010. "Antidepressant Drug Effects and Depression Severity: A Patient-Level Meta-Analysis." *Journal of the American Medical Association* 303 (1): 47–53. Accessed August 17, 2017. https://www.ncbi.nlm.nih.gov/pubmed/20051569.

Full Measure Staff. 2017. "Fake Science." *Full Measure News.* May 7. Accessed July 21, 2017. http://fullmeasure.news/news/cover-story/fake-science.

Ghosal, U.C., et al. 2017. "Small Intestinal Bacterial Overgrowth and Irritable Bowel Syndrome: A Bridge between Functional Organic Dichotomy." *Gut Liver* 11 (2): 196. Accessed August 17, 2017. https://www.ncbi.nlm.nih.gov/pubmed/28274108.

Goldhill, David. 2013. *Catastrophic Care: How American Health Care Killed My Father—And How We Can Fix It.* New York: Knopf Doubleday.

Grenny, Joseph, et al. 2008. "How to Have Influence." *MIT Sloan Management Review Magazine* 50 (1). Accessed August 17, 2017. http://sloanreview.mit.edu/article/how-to-have-influence/.

Gurven, Michael, and Hillard Kaplan. 2007. "Longevity among Hunter-Gatherers: A Cross-Cultural Examination." *Population and Development Review* 33 (2): 321-365. Accessed July 24, 2017. http://onlinelibrary.wiley.com/doi/10.1111/j.1728-4457.2007.00171.x/abstract.

Guyenet, Stephan. 2008. "Conflicts of Interest." *Whole Health Source Nutrition and Health Science.* August 28. Accessed July 24, 2017. http://wholehealthsource.blogspot.com/2008/08/conflict-of-interest.html.

Hartung, T. 2013. "Food for Thought: Look Back in Anger—What Clinical Studies Tell Us about Preclinical Work." *ALTEX* 30 (3): 275–291. Accessed August 17, 2017. https://www.ncbi.nlm.nih.gov/pmc/articles/PMC3790571/.

Henry, Amanda G., et al. 2010. "Microfossils in Calculus Demonstrate Consumption of Plants and Cooked Foods in Neanderthal Diets." *Proceedings of the National Academy of Sciences (PNAS)* 108 (2): 486–491. Accessed August 17, 2017. http://www.pnas.org/content/108/2/486.full.pdf.

Holt-Lunstad, Julianne, et al. 2010. "Social Relationships and Mortality Risk: A Meta-Analytic Review." *PLoS Medicine* 7 (7). Accessed July 24, 2017. https://doi.org/10.1371/journal.pmed.1000316.

Hyman, Mark. 2010. "Failure of Risk Factor Treatment for Chronic Disease." *Alternative Therapies* 16 (3): 60–3. Accessed August 17, 2017. https://www.ncbi.nlm.nih.gov/pubmed/20486626.

IMS Health. 2016. "IMS Health Study: U.S. Drug Spending Growth Reaches 8.5 Percent in 2015." *IMSHealth.com.* April 14. Accessed July 24, 2017. http://www.imshealth.com/en/about-us/news/ims-health-study-us-drug-spending-growth-reaches-8.5-percent-in-2015.

Ioannidis, John P.A. 2005. "Why Most Published Research Findings Are False." *PLoS Medicine* 2 (8): e124. Accessed July 24, 2017. http://journals.plos.org/plosmedicine/article?id=10.1371/journal.pmed.0020124.

Johns Hopkins University Partnership for Solutions. 2004. *Chronic Conditions: Making the Case for Ongoing Care.* Boston: Johns Hopkins University. Accessed July 24, 2017. http://www.partnershipforsolutions.org/DMS/files/chronicbook2004.pdf.

Kaplan, H., et al. 2017. "Coronary Atherosclerosis in Indigenous South American Tsimane: A Cross-Sectional Cohort Study." *Lancet* 389 (10080): 1730–1739. Accessed August 17, 2017. http://www.thelancet.com/journals/lancet/article/PIIS0140-6736(17)30752-3/fulltext.

Knutson, K.L., et al. 2010. "Trends in the Prevalence of Short Sleepers in the USA: 1975–2006." *Sleep* 33 (1): 37–45. Accessed August 17, 2017. https://www.ncbi.nlm.nih.gov/pubmed/20120619.

Kresser, Chris. 2013a. "50 Shades of Gluten (Intolerance)." *Chris Kresser: Let's Take Back Your Health—Starting Now.* April 23. Accessed August 17, 2017. https://chriskresser. com/50-shades-of-gluten-intolerance/.

—. 2013b. "What Causes Elevated LDL Particle Number?" *Chris Kresser: Let's Take Back Your Health—Starting Now.* May 3. Accessed July 24, 2017. https://chriskresser.com/ what-causes-elevated-ldl-particle-number/.

—. 2015. "Behind the Veil: Conflicts of Interest and Fraud in Medical Research." *Chris Kresser: Let's Take Back Your Health—Starting Now.* February 17. Accessed July 24, 2017. https://chriskresser. com/behind-the-veil-conflicts-of-interest-and-fraud-in-medical-research/.

—. 2016. "The Dangers of Proton Pump Inhibitors." *Chris Kresser: Let's Take Back Your Health—Starting Now.* June 14. Accessed August 17, 2017. https://chriskresser.com/ the-dangers-of-proton-pump-inhibitors/.

—. 2017. "Two Reasons Conventional Medicine Will Never Solve Chronic Disease." *Chris Kresser: Let's Take Back Your Health—Starting Now.* June 14. Accessed July 24, 2017. https:// chriskresser.com/two-reasons-conventional-medicine-will-never-solve-chronic-disease/.

Kresser Institute. 2017. Survey of Incoming Practitioners in the ADAPT Practitioner Training Program. April 2017.

LaMontagne, Christina. 2013. "Medical Bankruptcy Accounts for Majority of Personal Bankruptcies." *nerdwallet.* June 19. Accessed August 17, 2017. https://www.nerdwallet.com/blog/health/medical-bankruptcy/.

Levine, Hagai, et al. 2017. "Temporal Trends in Sperm Count: A Systematic Review and Meta-Regression Analysis." *Human Reproduction Update.* July 25, 2017. Accessed August 17, 2017. https://academic.oup.com/humupd/article/doi/10.1093/humupd/dmx022/4035689/Temporal-trends-in-sperm-count-a-systematic-review.

Levinson, Daniel. 2009. "How Grantees Manage Financial Conflicts of Interest in Research Funded by the National Institutes of Health." Department of Human Health and Services, Office of Inspector General. November 2009. Accessed August 19, 2017. https://oig.hhs.gov/oei/reports/oei-03-07-00700.pdf.

Lexchin, Joel. 2003. "Pharmaceutical Industry Sponsorship and Research Outcome and Quality: Systematic Review." *The BMJ* 326: 1167. Accessed August 17, 2017. http://www.bmj.com/content/326/7400/1167.

Loscalzo, J., et al. 2007. "Human Disease Classification in the Postgenomic Era: A Complex Systems Approach to Human Pathobiology." *Molecular Systems Biology* 3: 124. Accessed August 17, 2017. https://www.ncbi.nlm.nih.gov/pubmed/17625512.

Mensink, R.P., et al. 2003. "Effects of Dietary Fatty Acids and Carbohydrates on the Ration of Serum Total to HDL Cholesterol and on Serum Lipids and Apolipoproteins: A Meta-Analysis of 60 Controlled Trials." *American Journal of Clinical Nutrition* 77 (5): 1146–55. Accessed August 17, 2017. https://www.ncbi.nlm.nih.gov/pubmed/12716665.

Mirkarimi, K., et al. 2015. "Effect of Motivational Interviewing on a Weight Loss Program Based on the Protection Motivation Theory." *Iranian Red Crescent Medical Journal* 17 (6). Accessed August 17, 2017. https://www.ncbi.nlm.nih.gov/pubmed/26380106.

Möhlenkamp, S., et al. 2008. "Running: The Risk of Coronary Events: Prevalence and Prognostic Relevance of Coronary Atherosclerosis in Marathon Runners." *European Heart Journal* 29 (15): 1903–1910. Accessed August 17, 2017. https://www.ncbi.nlm.nih.gov/pubmed/18426850.

Munro, Dan. 2015. "U.S. Healthcare Spending on Track to Hit $10,000 Per Person This Year." *Forbes.com*. January 4. Accessed July 21, 2017. https://www.forbes.com/sites/danmunro/2015/01/04/u-s-healthcare-spending-on-track-to-hit-10000-per-person-this-year/#7530de2e6dea.

National Center for Chronic Disease Prevention and Health Promotion (NCCDPHP). 2016. "At a Glance 2016." *CDC.gov*. Accessed July 21, 2017. https://www.cdc.gov/chronicdisease/resources/publications/aag/nccdphp.htm.

—. 2016. "Chronic Diseases: The Leading Causes of Death and Disability in the United States." *CDC.gov*. Accessed July 21, 2017. https://www.cdc.gov/chronicdisease/overview/index.htm.

National Institute of Environmental Health Sciences (NIEHS). 2012. "Autoimmune Diseases." *National Institutes of Health U.S. Department of Health and Human Services.* November. Accessed July 24, 2017. https://www.niehs.nih.gov/health/materials/auto-immune_diseases_508.pdf.

National Institutes of Health (NIH). 2017. "Rates of New Diagnosed Cases of Type 1 and Type 2 Diabetes on the Rise among Children, Teens." April 13. Accessed August 17, 2017. https://www.nih.gov/news-events/news-releases/rates-new-diagnosed-cases-type-1-type-2-diabetes-rise-among-children-teens.

Nikrahan, G.R., et al. 2016. "Effects of Positive Psychology Interventions on Risk Biomarkers in Coronary Patients: A Randomized, Wait-List Controlled Pilot Trial." *Psychosomatics* 57 (4): 359–68. Accessed August 17, 2017. https://www.ncbi.nlm.nih.gov/pubmed/27129358.

Olshansky, S. Jay, et al. 2005. "A Potential Decline in Life Expectancy in the United States in the 21st Century." *The New England Journal of Medicine* 352: 1138–1145. Accessed August 17, 2017. http://www.nejm.org/doi/full/10.1056/NEJMsr043743#t=article.

Open Science Collaborators. 2015. "Psychology: Estimating the Reproducibility of Psychological Science." *Science* 349 (6251). Accessed August 17, 2017. http://science.sciencemag.org/content/349/6251/aac4716.

Petterson, Stephen M., et al. 2012. "Projecting US Primary Care Physician Workforce Needs: 2010–2025." *Annals of Family Medicine* 10 (6): 503–509. Accessed August 17, 2017. http://www.annfammed.org/content/10/6/503.abstract.

Rappaport, S.M. 2016. "Genetic Factors Are Not the Major Cause of Chronic Diseases." *PLoS One* 11 (4). Accessed July 21, 2017. https://www.ncbi.nlm.nih.gov/pubmed/27105432.

Rhoades, D.R., et al. 2001. "Speaking and Interruptions during Primary Care Office Visits." *Family Medicine* 33 (7): 528–32. Accessed August 17, 2017. https://www.ncbi.nlm.nih.gov/pubmed/11456245.

Schimpff, Stephen C. 2015. *Fixing the Primary Care Crisis: Reclaiming the Patient-Doctor Relationship and Returning Healthcare Decisions to You and Your Doctor.* CreateSpace Independent Publishing Platform.

Schneider, Eric C., et al. 2017. "Mirror, Mirror 2017: International Comparison Reflects Flaws and Opportunities for Better U.S. Health Care." *The Commonwealth Fund.* Accessed August 17, 2017. http://www.commonwealthfund.org/publications/fund-reports/2017/jul/mirror-mirror-international-comparisons-2017.

Seife, C. 2015. "Research Misconduct Identified by the US Food and Drug Administration: Out of Sight, Out of Mind, Out of the Peer-Reviewed Literature." *Journal of the American Medical Association: Internal Medicine* 175 (4): 567. Accessed August 17, 2017. https://www.ncbi.nlm.nih.gov/pubmed/25664866.

Siri-Tarino, P.W., et al. 2010. "Meta-Analysis of Prospective Cohort Studies Evaluating the Association of Saturated Fat with Cardiovascular Disease." *American Journal of Clinical Nutrition* 91 (3): 535–46. Accessed August 17, 2017. https://www.ncbi.nlm.nih.gov/pubmed/20071648.

Slattery, J., et al. 2016. "Enteric Ecosystem Disruption in Autism Spectrum Disorder: Can the Microbiota and Macrobiota be Restored?" *Current Pharmaceutical Design* 40: 6107–6121. Accessed August 17, 2017. https://www.ncbi.nlm.nih.gov/pubmed/27592717.

Smith, Ronald S. 2010. *Cytokines and Depression: How Your Immune System Causes Depression.* eBook. Accessed August 17, 2017. http://www.cytokines-and-depression.com/chapter7.html.

Smith, R., et al. 2014. "Should Journals Stop Publishing Research Funded by the Drug Industry?" *BMJ* 348. Accessed July 21, 2017. https://www.ncbi.nlm.nih.gov/pubmed/24423895.

Snyderman, R., and J. Langheier. 2006. "Prospective Health Care: The Second Transformation of Medicine." *Genome Biology* 7 (2): 104. Accessed August 17, 2017. https://www.ncbi.nlm.nih.gov/pubmed/16522218.

Starfield, Barbara. 2000. "Is US Health Really the Best in the World?" *Journal of the American Medical Association* 284 (4): 483. Accessed August 17, 2017. https://www.jhsph.edu/research/centers-and-institutes/johns-hopkins-primary-care-policy-center/Publications_PDFs/A154.pdf.

The Physician's Foundation. 2016. *2016 Survey of America's Physicians: Practice Patterns & Perspectives.* The Physicians Foundation. Accessed July 24, 2017. http://www.physiciansfoundation.org/uploads/default/Biennial_Physician_Survey_2016.pdf.

Trowell, H.C., and D.P. Burkitt. 1981. *Western Diseases: Their Emergence and Prevention.* Boston: Harvard University Press.

Tziatzios, G., et al. 2017. "Is Small Intestinal Bacterial Overgrowth Involved in the Pathogenesis of Functional Dyspepsia?" *Medical Hypotheses* 106: 26–32. Accessed August 17, 2017. https://www.ncbi.nlm.nih.gov/pubmed/28818267.

Van Cleave, J., et al. 2010. "Dynamics of Obesity and Chronic Health Conditions among Children and Youth." *Journal of the American Medical Association* 303 (7): 623–630. Accessed August 17, 2017. https://www.ncbi.nlm.nih.gov/pubmed/20159870.

Wahls, Terry. 2014. *The Wahls Protocol: A Radical New Way to Treat All Chronic Autoimmune Conditions Using Paleo Principles.* New York: Avery.

Williamson, S.H., et al. 2007. "Localising Recent Adaptive Evolution in the Human Genome." *PLOS Genetics* 3 (6): E90. Accessed July 24, 2017. http://journals.plos.org/plosgenetics/article?id=10.1371/journal.pgen.0030090.

Wright, K.P., Jr., et al. 2013. "Entrainment of the Human Circadian Clock to the Natural Light-Dark Cycle." *Current Biology* 23 (16): 1554–8. Accessed August 17, 2017. https://www.ncbi.nlm.nih.gov/pubmed/23910656.

Yamagishi, K., et al. 2010. "Dietary Intake of Saturated Fatty Acids and Mortality from Cardiovascular Disease in Japanese: The Japan Collaborative Cohort Study for Evaluation of Cancer Risk (JACC) Study." *American Journal of Clinical Nutrition* 92 (4): 759–65. Accessed August 17, 2017. https://www.ncbi.nlm.nih.gov/pubmed/20685950.

Yawn, B., et al. 2003. "Time Use During Acute and Chronic Illness Visits to a Family Physician." *Family Practice* 20 (4): 474-7. Accessed August 17, 2017. https://www.ncbi.nlm.nih.gov/pubmed/12876124.

Zablotsky, Benjamin, et al. 2015. "Estimated Prevalence of Autism and Other Developmental Disabilities Following Question-naire Changes in the 2014 National Health Interview Survey." *National Health Statistics Report* 87: 1-20. Accessed August 18, 2017. https://www.ncbi.nlm.nih.gov/pubmed/26632847.

Zhao, Yafu, and William Encinosa. 2008. "Gastroesophageal Reflux Disease (GERD) Hospitalizations in 1998 and 2005." *H-CUP Statistical Brief* (Agency for Healthcare Research and Quality, Healthcare Cost and Utilization Project). Accessed July 24, 2017. https://www.hcup-us.ahrq.gov/reports/statbriefs/sb44.pdf.

Ziv-Gal, Ayelet, et al. 2016. "The Effects of In Utero Bisphenol A Exposure on Reproductive Capacity in Several Generations of Mice." *Toxicology and Applied Pharmacology* 284 (3): 354-362. Accessed August 17, 2017. https://www.ncbi.nlm.nih.gov/pubmed/25771130.

ABOUT THE AUTHOR

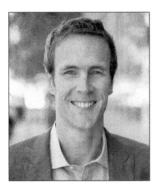 **Chris Kresser, M.S., L.Ac**, is the founder of Kresser Institute, the co-director of the California Center for Functional Medicine, the creator of ChrisKresser. com, and the *New York Times* best-selling author of *The Paleo Cure*. Known for his research uncovering myths in modern medicine and providing proven natural health solutions, Chris was named one of the 100 most influential people in health and fitness by Greatist.com (along with Michelle Obama, Dr. Oz, Dr. Weil, Deepak Chopra, and Dr. Mercola). His blog is one of the top-ranked natural health websites in the world. Chris lives in Berkeley, California, with his family.